Neurodevelopment and Neurodevelopmental Disorder

Edited by Michael Fitzgerald

Published in London, United Kingdom

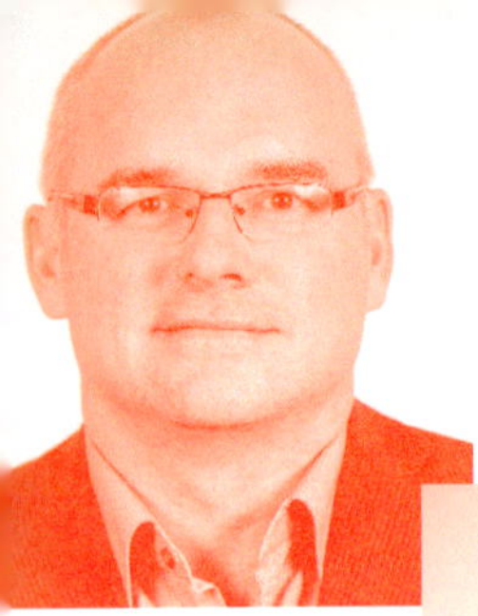
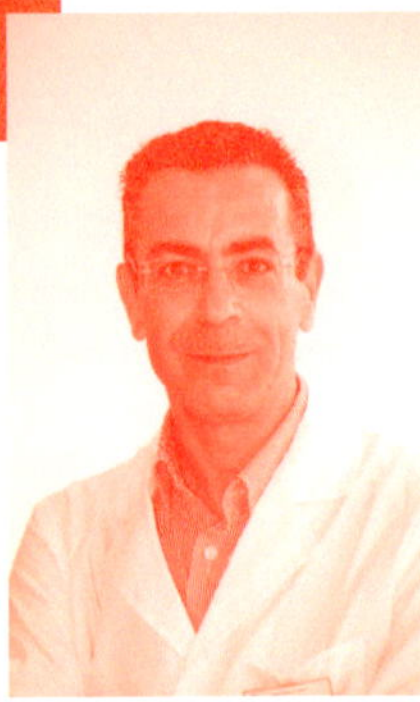
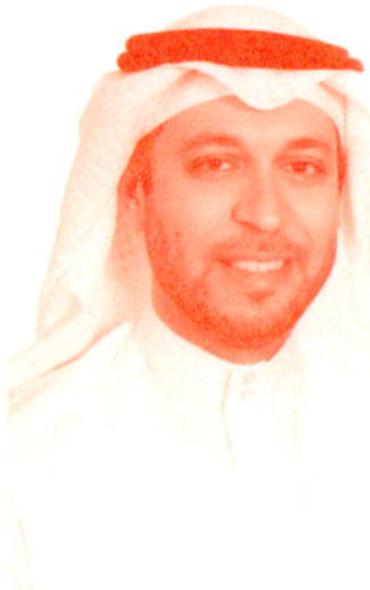
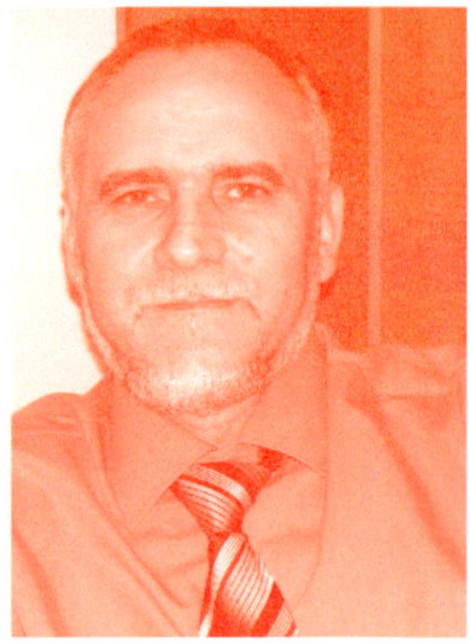
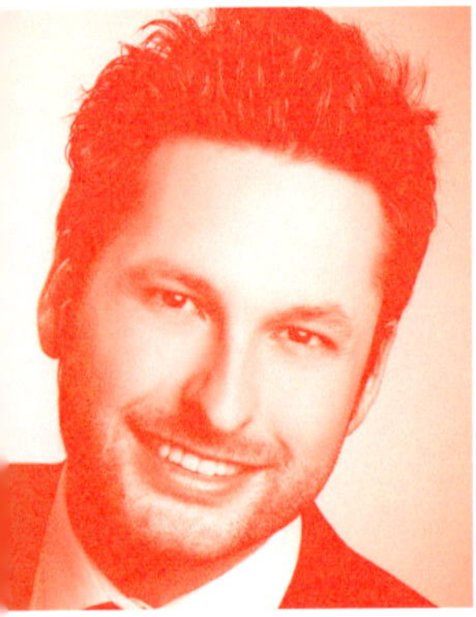
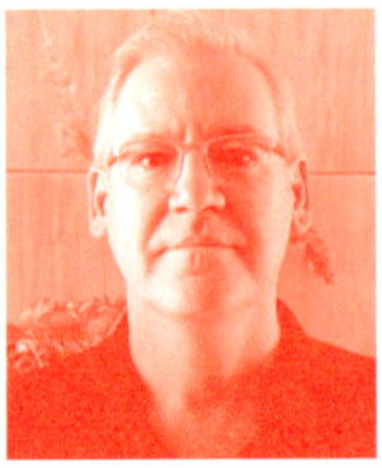
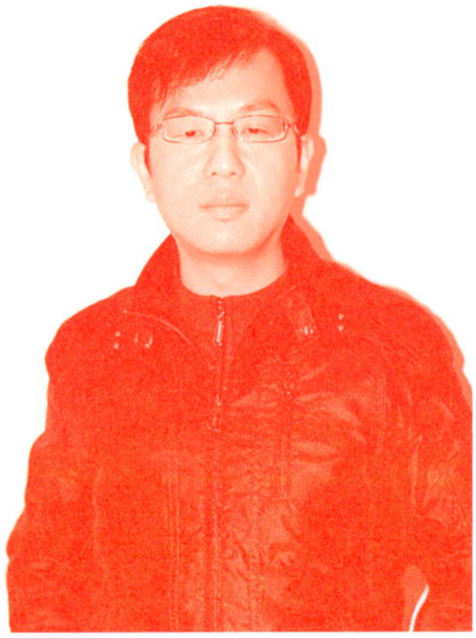

IntechOpen

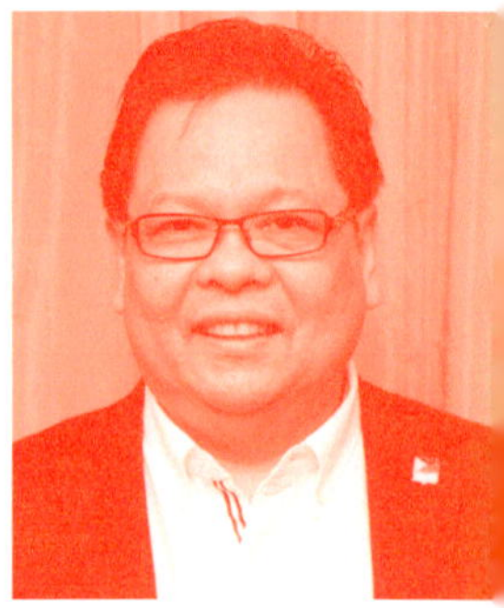
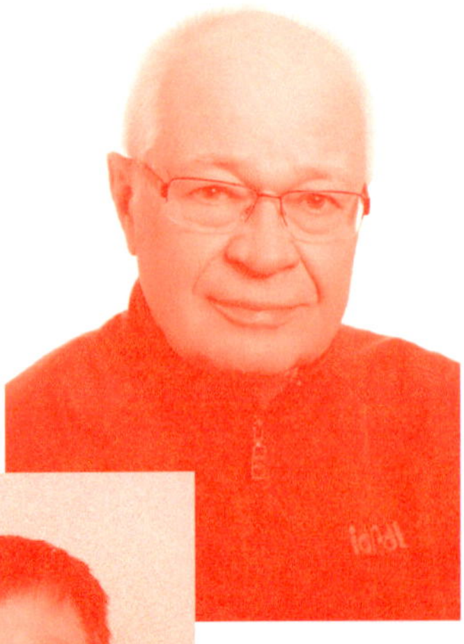
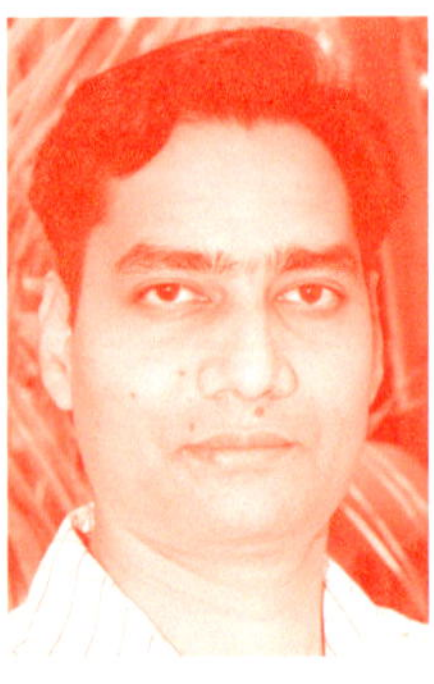
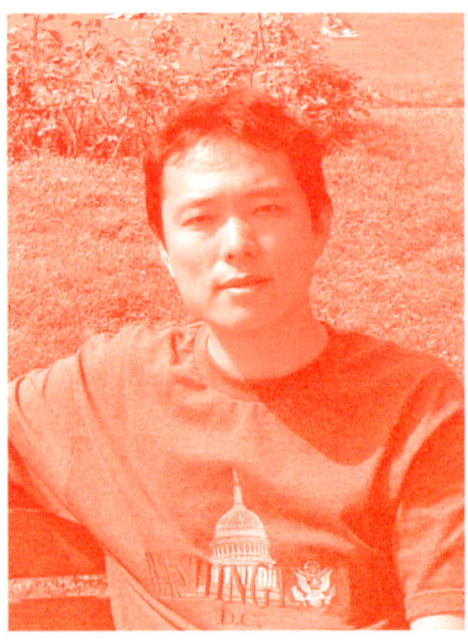
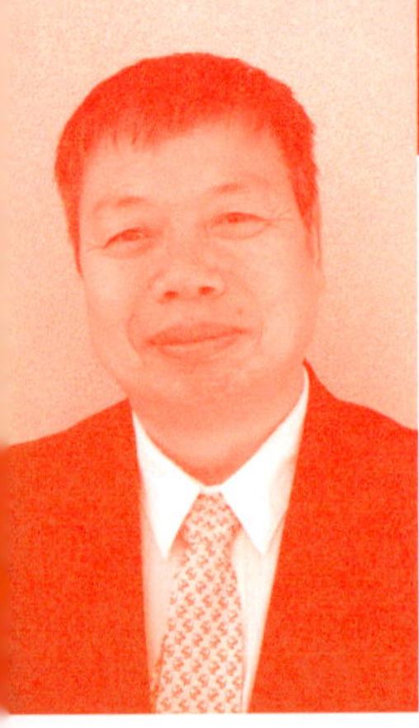
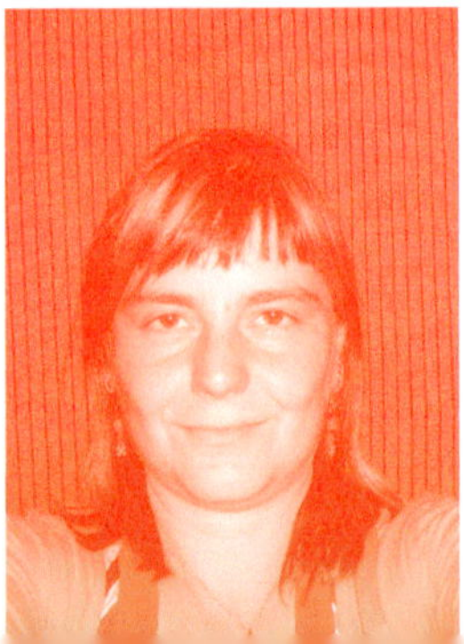

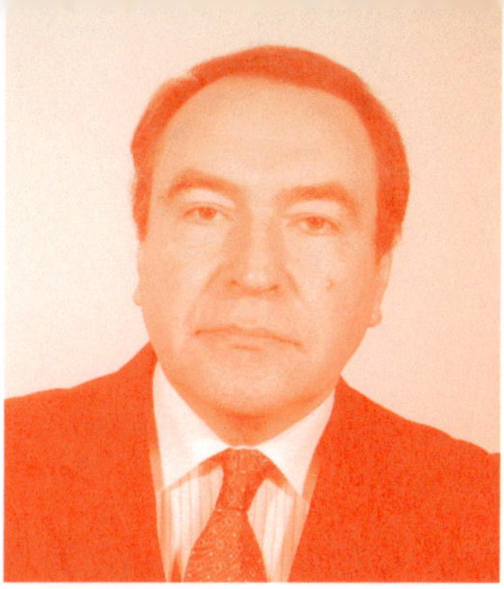
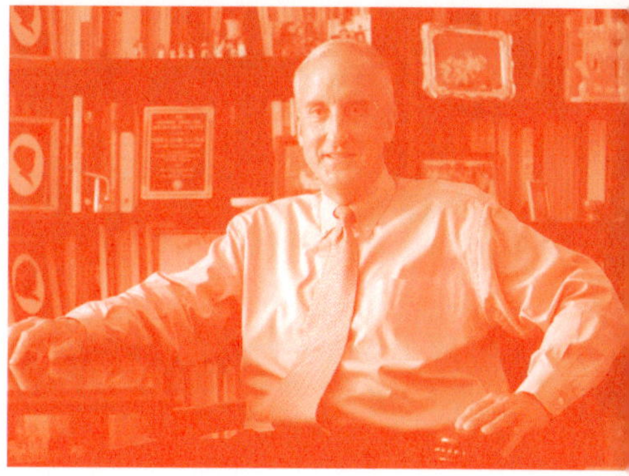
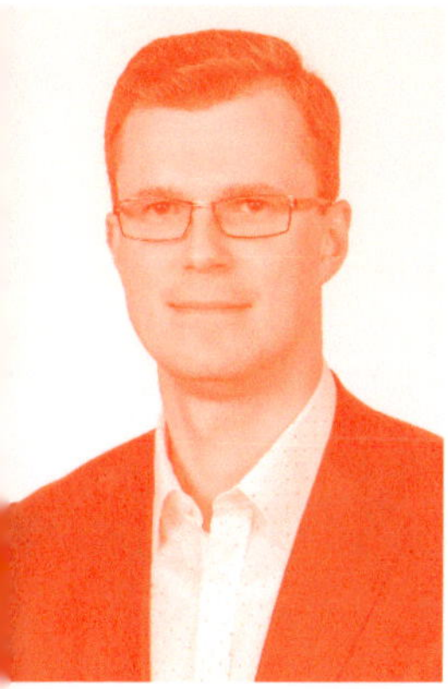
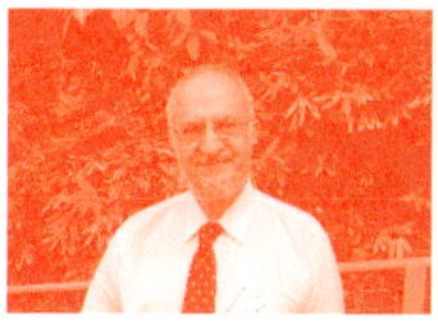
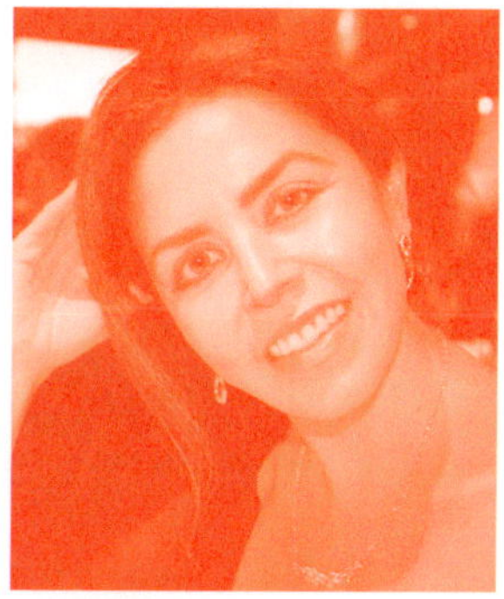

Supporting open minds since 2005

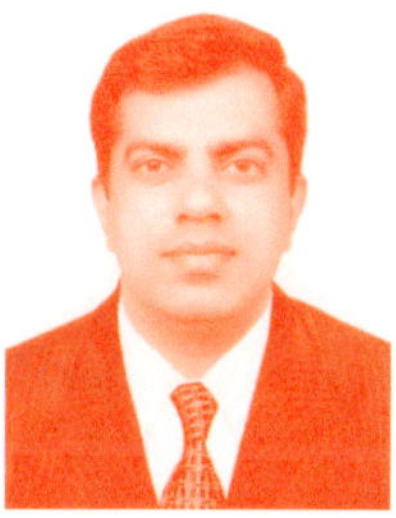
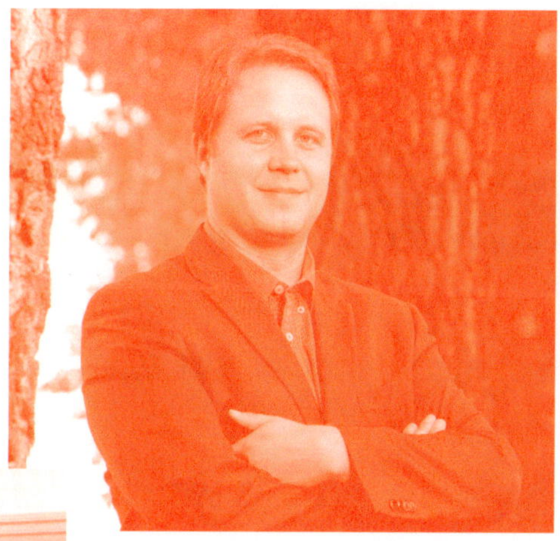
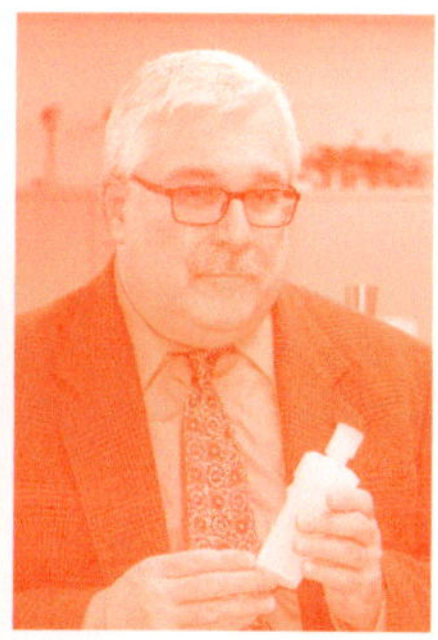
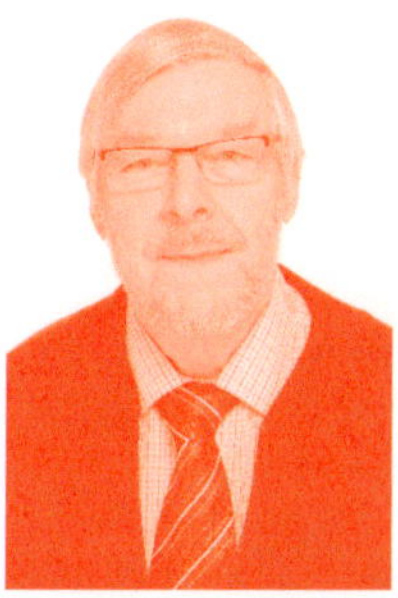
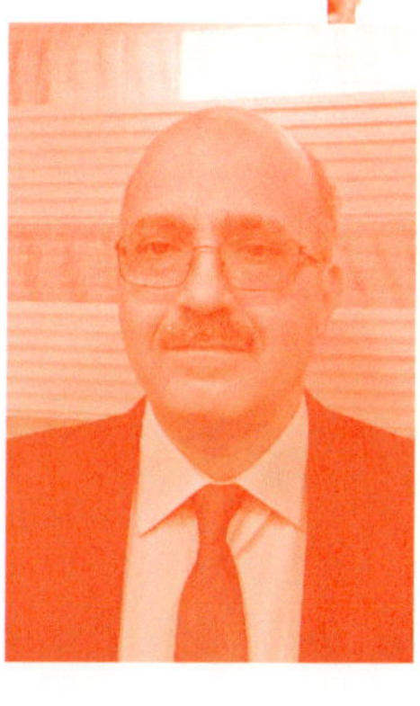
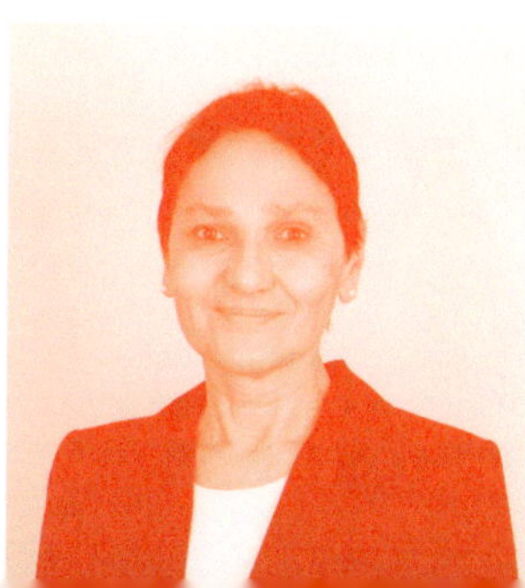
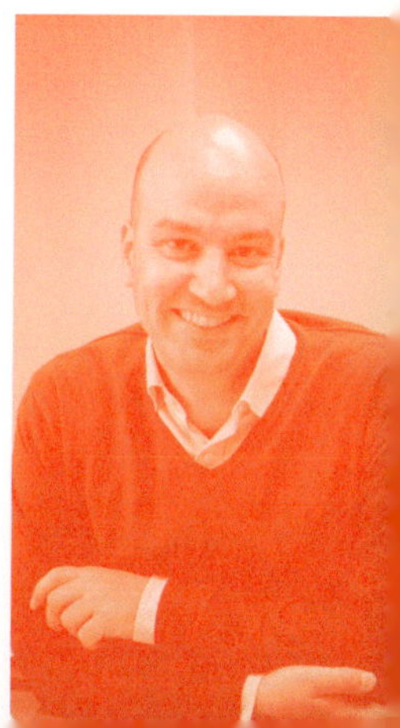

Neurodevelopment and Neurodevelopmental Disorder
http://dx.doi.org/10.5772/intechopen.78797
Edited by Michael Fitzgerald

Part of IntechOpen Book Series: Physiology, Volume 6
Book Series Editor: Angel Catala

Contributors
Boulenouar Mesraoua, Dirk Deleu, Hassan Al Hail, Naim Haddad, Gayane Melykian, Ali A. Asadi-Pooya, , Covanis Athanasios, Musab Ali, Delia Marina Podea, Romina-Teodora Moldovan, Laura Cristina Popa, Bobbie Koen, Hagit Friedman, Marina Soloveichick, Amir Kushnir, Hava Kasher, Caroline Barmatz, Omer Bar-Yosef, Marwa Saleh, Aya Adel, Michael Fitzgerald, Marco Antonio Mendoza Parra, Elodie Mathieux, Albert Ribes-Zamora

First published in London, United Kingdom, 2019 by IntechOpen
IntechOpen is the global imprint of INTECHOPEN LIMITED, registered in England and Wales, registration number: 11086078, 7th floor, 10 Lower Thames Street, London, EC3R 6AF, United Kingdom
Printed in Croatia

British Library Cataloguing-in-Publication Data
A catalogue record for this book is available from the British Library

Additional hard and PDF copies can be obtained from orders@intechopen.com

Neurodevelopment and Neurodevelopmental Disorder
Edited by Michael Fitzgerald
p. cm.
Print ISBN 978-1-78923-825-9
Online ISBN 978-1-78923-826-6
eBook (PDF) ISBN 978-1-78984-371-2
ISSN 2631-8261

For EU product safety concerns:
IN TECH d.o.o., Prolaz Marije Krucifikse Kozulić 3, 51000 Rijeka, Croatia, info@intechopen.com or visit our website at intechopen.com.

IntechOpen Book Series
Physiology
Volume 6

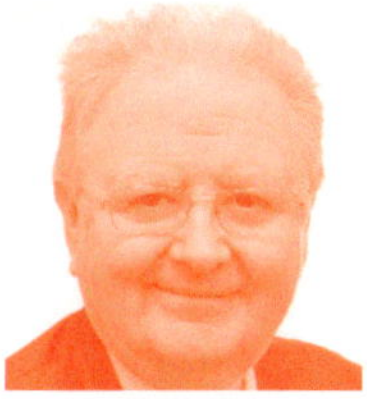

Professor Michael Fitzgerald was the first Professor of Child and Adolescent Psychiatry in Ireland. Specialising in Autism Spectrum Disorders (ASDs), he has diagnosed more than 5000 persons with ASDs. He has written many peer-reviewed publications and authored, co-authored and co-edited 34 books that have been translated into Japanese, Dutch and Polish. Professor Simon Baron-Cohen of the University of Cambridge described one of Dr. Fitzgerald's books on autism as *"the best book on autism"* and described him as an *"exceptional scholar."* Dr. Fitzgerald has lectured extensively throughout the world including at The Royal Society/British Academy and the British Library in London. He was the overall winner of the "Excellence in Psychiatry" award in 2017 and was nominated as one of the top four psychiatrists by Hospital Professional News Ireland – Top 100 Professionals in Ireland 2017.

Editor of Volume 6: Professor M. Fitzgerald
Department of Psychiatry, Trinity College,
Dublin 2, Ireland

Book Series Editor: Angel Catala
National University of La Plata, Argentina

Scope of the Series

Modern physiology requires a comprehensive understanding of the integration of tissues and organs throughout the mammalian body, including the expression, structure, and function of molecular and cellular components. While a daunting task, learning is facilitated by our identification of common, effective signaling pathways employed by nature to sustain life. As a main example, the cellular interplay between intracellular Ca2 increases and changes in plasma membrane potential is integral to coordinating blood flow, governing the exocytosis of neurotransmitters and modulating genetic expression. Further, in this manner, understanding the systemic interplay between the cardiovascular and nervous systems has now become more important than ever as human populations age and mechanisms of cellular oxidative signaling are utilized for sustaining life. Altogether, physiological research enables our identification of clear and precise points of transition from health to development of multi-morbidity during the inevitable aging process (e.g., diabetes, hypertension, chronic kidney disease, heart failure, age-related macular degeneration; cancer). With consideration of all organ systems (e.g., brain, heart, lung, liver; gut, kidney, eye) and the interactions thereof, this Physiology Series will address aims of resolve (1) Aging physiology and progress of chronic diseases (2) Examination of key cellular pathways as they relate to calcium, oxidative stress, and electrical signaling & (3) how changes in plasma membrane produced by lipid peroxidation products affects aging physiology

Contents

Preface

Neurodevelopmental disorders are the new psychiatry. One of the tragedies of the twentieth century, particularly in child and adolescent psychiatry and to a lesser extent in adult psychiatry and psychology, was the tradition of blaming families, especially mothers, for psychiatric problems. Tragically we had, 'schizophrenic mothers' as causes of schizophrenia and 'refrigerator mothers' as causes of autism.

These false theories caused untold distress to mothers and families. It does appear to me that attachment theorists could be in danger, using a different theory, of repeating some of these same errors and causing more unnecessary guilt among mothers.

At a clinical level I have seen many children described as having attachment disorders, who actually have classic Asperger syndrome. Asperger's is still listed in the *International Statistical Classification of Diseases* (ICD-10), but has been incorporated into autism spectrum disorders in the *Diagnostic and Statistical Manual of Mental Disorders, Fifth Edition* (DSM-5).

Over many years, I have observed how it is almost impossible for professionals trained in the theories of Sigmund Freud and John Bowlby to take on board the neurodevelopmental disorders of attention deficit hyperactivity disorder (ADHD), autism, Asperger syndrome, and so on.

Other disorders, including learning disability, bipolar disorder, and schizophrenia, are now recognised as neurodevelopmental. These three cause less difficulty for clinicians, although Asperger syndrome is often misdiagnosed as bipolar disorder or borderline personality disorder or schizophrenia.

All of these neurodevelopmental conditions overlap to a greater or lesser extent. They are not separate categories, that is, they are not categorised in narrow diagnostic 'boxes'. They are best seen along overlapping dimensional lines.

It is widely agreed that the current classifications in psychiatry are unsatisfactory. People have been aware for some time of the overlap between bipolar and schizophrenia, in relation to the psychotic spectrum [1]. I have quite a number of patients on the autism spectrum who developed psychosis in adult life, or indeed sooner. Overlap of conditions is extremely common and each element of the overlap must be identified and treated.

All of these disorders have major genetic underpinnings. Indeed some genetic findings overlap between these developmental disorders with other non-overlapping findings.

The future of psychiatry will be neurodevelopmental in large measure. Psychiatrists will focus on these conditions, while psychotherapists, counsellors and psychologists will treat mild psychiatric conditions with psychotherapeutic interventions.

We have a long way to go before we achieve the vision set forth by Thomas Insel, former director of the National Institute of Mental Health in the United States (NIMH), who stated that future diagnosis in psychiatry should be based on biomarkers, neuroimaging and laboratory tests [2–4]. This is only aspirational at this point.

The first chapter of this book sets out the future of psychiatry in relation to neurodevelopmental disorders and what is basically a new understanding of psychiatry in recent decades. Other chapters address topics such as the early recognition of schizophrenia, early intervention for babies at risk of neurodevelopmental disorders, epilepsy, and the genetics of ataxia telangiectasia. Finally, this book examines the complex issue of systems biology and neurodevelopment.

M. Fitzgerald
Professor,
Department of Psychiatry,
Trinity College,
Ireland

References

[1] Fitzgerald M. Schizophrenia and autism, clinical overlap and difference. Clinical Neuropsychiatry. 2012;**10**(4):171-176

[2] McCarthy SE, Makarov V, Kirov G, Addington AM, et al. Micro duplications of 16p11.2 are associated with schizophrenia. Nature Genetics. 2009;**41**:1223-1227

[3] Craddock N, Mynors-Wallis L. Psychiatric diagnosis: Impersonal, imperfect and important. British Journal of Psychiatry. 2014;**204**(2):93-95

[4] Craddock N, Owen M. The Kraepelian dichotomy- going, going, but still not gone. British Journal of Psychiatry. 2010;**196**(2):92-95

Section 1

The Future of Psychiatry is Neurodevelopmental

Chapter 1

The Future of Psychiatry and Neurodevelopmental Disorders: A Paradigm Shift

Michael Fitzgerald

Abstract

A paradigm shift is now taking place in psychiatry with the emphasis on neurodevelopmental disorders with a neurobiologic emphasis and early onset including autism, ADHD, learning disability, schizophrenia and bipolar disorder. This paradigm superseded the attachment paradigm of the second half of the twentieth century with so many misguided theories such as, "blaming the mother"—the so-called refrigerated mother and the schizophrenogenic mother. The new paradigm allows more focused treatment interventions.

Keywords: neurodevelopmental disorders, autism, attachment disorders, neurobiology

1. Introduction

The future of psychiatry is neurodevelopmental. One of the tragedies of the twentieth century, more particularly in child and adolescent psychiatry, is the tradition of blaming families and particularly mothers for psychiatric problems. Tragically, we had "schizophrenogenic mothers" as "causes" of schizophrenia and "refrigerated mothers" as "causes" of autism. Even more recently, tragically, John Bowlby [1], in discussing "causal factors" in relation to autism, mentioned "inappropriate mothering". This is another mother-blaming idea. The current understanding of these disorders, intellectual disability, ADHD, autism, Asperger's syndrome, tics, etc., is a neurodevelopmental disorder with schizophrenia and bipolar disorder also being neurodevelopmental, and all have significant neurobiological inputs. Some personality disorders should also be considered as being on the neurodevelopmental spectrum. The neurodevelopmental trajectory will include the addition of more neurodevelopmental disorders, e.g., bipolar, schizophrenia and depression as the person gets older.

2. Adult autism

All diagnoses of autism have to take a developmental history from childhood, which will include persistent deficits in social communication and social interaction from the early developmental period, as well as restricted, repetitive patterns of behaviour causing clinically significant impairment in functioning (American Psychiatric Association [2]). The problem with adult autism diagnosis will include getting a relatively early history from an informant which may be a parent or other, the problem of camouflaging because of treatment or just life experience which makes it more difficult to diagnose the adult with autism. They may have learned about eye contact, etc. School reports or home videos sometimes help. They will often present with comorbidities, for example, depression, (70%), anxiety (40%), attention deficit disorder or psychosis. Mazefsky and White [3] "caution against excessive reliance on ADOS (Autism Diagnostic Observation Scale), Lord et al. [4] for diagnosis".

3. Autism and schizophrenia

Schizophrenia and bipolar disorder are now seen as neurodevelopmental disorders with a widening of the neurodevelopmental spectrum.

Evans [5] states that the diagnosis of "schizophrenia, psychosis and autism in children, were largely interchangeable during the 1940s and 1950s" [6]. They were described as separate by Kolvin et al. [7]. This view was not supported [8].

According to Scull [9], Steven Hyman, the former director of NIMH stated that DSM 5 "was totally wrong in the way it's authors could not have imagined. So in fact, what they produced was an absolute scientific nightmare. Many people who got one diagnosis got five diagnoses, but they did not have five diseases—they have one underlying condition". Thomas Insel [9], who was also the director of the NIMH stated that DSM 5 showed "a lack of validity ... as long as the research community takes DSM 5 to be a bible, we will never make progress. People think that everything has to match DSM 5 criteria, but what you know ... biology never the book, and he went on to point out that in future the NIMH would be, "re-orientating into research away from DSM 5 categories ... patients with mental illness deserve better". Indeed, the NIMHS, under their director, Insel, gave up on this and aimed at a transdiagnostic study of psychiatric problems, and further studies should be based on biomarkers, neuroimaging and laboratory tests. This is a good aspiration and research efforts are being made in that direction. Clearly, Hyman and Insel were absolutely correct. He [9] proposed Research Domain Criteria to collect "genomic, cellular, imaging, social and behavioural information", and he also recommended focusing on the brain and "connectopathies". Thomas Insel noted that psychiatrists "actually believe, (that their diagnoses) are real, but there's no reality. They are just constructs". The first step is to analyse the huge spectrum of empathy and diagnosis.

Rutter [10] states that "the concept of autism as a variety of schizophrenia is very probably wrong". The real answer is that they overlap and are not watertight categories. Rutter [11] stated that "infantile autism is not anything to do with schizophrenia, is not primarily a disorder of social relationship". This is incorrect because they do overlap and autism is primarily a disorder of social relationships. Sullivan et al. [8] point out that "ASD, schizophrenia and bipolar disorder share common aetiological factors". This would be supported by Abel [12] who points out that "it has been suggested that, (as for common genetic variants), many of the candidate genes identified may not be coding for schizophrenia per se, but for a broader construct such as psychosis, or neurocognitive deficits which occur in schizophrenia and other conditions". Rapaport et al. [13] states that many individually rare genetic abnormalities affect common pathways containing hundreds of genes that affect neuronal development and regulation. Carroll et al. [14] point out that some of the specific genetic loci implicated encode proteins, such as neurexins and neuroligins, which function in synaptic development and plasticity and therefore represent a common biological pathway for disorders. Fatemi [15] points out the pathological involvement of Reelin gene or its protein product in autism and schizophrenia.

Reelin is a glycoprotein that helps guide brain development in an orderly fashion [15]. Fatemi [15] notes that Reelin deficits may cause abnormal corticogenesis and alter synaptic plasticity. In addition, Burbach et al. [16] note that contact in associated protein affects receptor/signalling units and are thought to mediate neuron-glial cell interactions, neuron migration and dendritic orientation. Contactin is a member of the neurexin family, and there are deletions and disruptions in neurexin 1 in autism and schizophrenia.

Rutter [17] points out that "adult schizophrenia is rare in both parents and brothers and sisters of autistic children". This is incorrect. Stone et al. [18] pointed out that there's evidence that parental diagnosis of schizophrenia was associated with elevated rates of autism offspring. Rapaport et al. [13] points out that familial schizophrenia like psychosis is a risk factor for "narrowly defined autism".

Both autism and schizophrenia can show formal thought disorder with poverty of content, illogical and loose associations. Solomon et al. [19] pointed out that when patients with first episode psychosis were compared to patients with ASD, they showed problems with semantics, syntax and coherence, although these deficits are more severe in ASD. They also noted that social interactional deficits are part of both conditions. Both have theory of mind deficits and problems with eye to eye gaze. In addition, they both have problems reading emotions from faces. Chris Frith [20] points out that "social withdrawal, stereotyped behaviour, and lack of communication are all typical features of childhood autism and chronic 'negative' schizophrenia". He emphasised mentalisation deficits in schizophrenia, which also occur in autism. In fact, they both show a disturbed sense of self. In comparison with schizophrenia, persons with autism show greater problems in reading faces, greater poverty of speech, as well as content and more perseveration of language, including echolalia and pronominal reversal, and more problems with set shifting and preservation of sameness. In comparison with autism, persons with schizophrenia show greater illogicality of thought, show more positive symptoms of psychosis, have mostly later onset (different from autism), run a more elapsing remitting course, show less stereotyped and repetitive behaviour, show less resistance to change, show less challenging behaviour as on an in-patient ward and show more jumping to conclusions.

Craddock and Owen [21] discuss a gradient of neurodevelopmental psychopathology from mental retardation to autism to schizophrenia to schizoaffective disorder to bipolar disorder. Nevertheless, the developmental process underlying these similar end points in autism and schizophrenia may be very different. Sporn et al. [22] suggest that "autistic behaviour may be a non-specific response to a variety of early developmental insults, and thus pre-morbid PDD (Pervasive Developmental Disorder) features in early onset schizophrenia may be an exaggeration of neurodevelopmental abnormalities seen in adult schizophrenia" and that "autism may reflect a separate additive risk factor for schizophrenia with very early onset". Certainly, psychotic risk factors are very similar to autistic symptoms, as is the case with schizotaxia, schizotypal personality disorder and schizoid personality disorder.

Rutter [23] states that delusions and hallucinations "are quite rare in autistic children, even when they reach adolescence and early adult life". This has not been my clinical experience, having diagnosed about 5000 children and adults and currently being involved with over 100 persons with autism in in-patient and out-patient settings.

Simple schizophrenia Kolb [24] is simply autism spectrum disorder. In my view, the so-called simple schizophrenia involves a disturbance of emotion, disturbance of interest, disturbance of activity, impoverishment of personality, shallowness of emotions and eccentricities. This would be classical high-functioning autism or what was called Asperger's syndrome in former classifications ICD 10 [25]. This is currently being updated.

Kanner [26] was correct when he pointed out that "the extreme isolation from people ... infantile autism bears so close a resemblance to schizophrenic withdrawal that the relationship between the two conditions deserves serious consideration". Of course other times, he described them as very separate. Asperger [27] pointed out that "the schizophrenic patient seems to show progressive loss of contact, the children we diagnose (now called Asperger's syndrome), lack contact from the start". The problem here is that some of the patients with autism do follow this pattern, but others have regressive autism, where they develop normally and then regress with loss of language, etc. I've seen this occurring up to 3 or 4 years of age.

Rutter [11] states that "the social class of parents of autistic children is most unlike that of the parents of schizophrenics. A high proportion of the parents of autistic children are of above average intelligence and superior socio-economic states". This is incorrect, as shown by Gillberg and Schumann [28]. In my clinical practice, I constantly see patients from every social class with autism and observe schizophrenia, bipolar disorder, etc. in their family histories.

4. Prevalence

Using narrow criteria of autism ADI-R, etc., Baird et al. [29] found a prevalence of 25 per 10,000, but when the broader autism spectrum criterium was used, a prevalence of 116 per 10,000 was found. This unfortunately means that over three quarters of the persons with autism in the community have what I would call "real" autism or clinical autism (autism spectrum disorder) and were missed by these narrow-based instruments. Currently, the prevalence of autism is 1/59 CDC and 1/37 males [30].

5. Differential diagnosis

See **Table 1** attached.

6. Tics, obsessive compulsive disorder and ASD

Canitano et al. [31] showed that 22% of ASDs presented with tic disorder, but there was a "difficulty in discriminating complex tics and OCD symptoms, and ASD symptoms". Nevertheless, the overlap between neurodevelopmental disorders is consistent. This equates with clinical experience and clinical reality. Maybe we need a subcategory called ASD plus tics and another category ASD without tics, another category with tics with ADHD and another category tics without ADHD, tics without OCD, etc. Stein [32] notes the overlap between autism, tics and stereotypic movement disorder. There is considerable neurobiological data in relation to OCD spectrum disorder. Stein [32] again emphasises the "possibly overlapping phenomenological and neurobiological features". Stein [32] points out that "there is increasing evidence that a sub-set of OCD may be genetically related to Tourette's Disorder, manifests with tics or OCD and involving both the serotonin or dopamine systems and the basal ganglia". Meir et al. [33] showed that "individuals diagnosed with OCD displayed a nearly four-fold higher risk to be diagnosed with ASD in later life" and that "the high co-morbidity sequential risk and shared familial risks between OCD and ASD's are suggestive of partially shared etiological mechanism". It would appear then that some neurosis (OCD) could be neurodevelopmental in origin, at least partly. This again shows the lack of sharp delineation between psychiatric diagnoses.

Asperger syndrome (DSM-IV) diagnostic criteria	Impairment in use of eye-to-eye gaze, facial expression, body postures	Failure to develop peer relationships to develop-mental level	Lack of spontaneous seeking to share enjoyment	Lack of social and emotional reciprocity	pre-occupation with one or more stereotyped pattern of interest	Inflexible adherence to specific non-functional routines or rituals	Stereotyped and repetitive motor mannerisms	Persistent pre-occupation with parts of objects	Clinically significant impairment in social or occupational functioning	No clinically significant delay in language development	No clinically significant delay in cognitive development or self-help skills
Schizoid personality in childhood		Yes	Yes	Yes	Yes	Yes			Yes	Yes	Yes
Obsessive compulsive personality disorder			Yes, often	Yes, often	Yes	Yes			Yes	Yes	Yes
Schizotypal disorder		Yes	Yes	Yes	Yes, sometimes				Yes	Yes	Yes
Avoidant personality disorder	Yes	Yes	Yes	Yes		Yes			Yes	Yes	Yes

Table 1.
Differential diagnosis of neurodevelopmental disorders (Asperger's syndrome).

7. Autism and ADHD

There is a very high comorbidity between autism and ADHD. Child psychiatric disorders have a comorbidity more than expected by chance [34]. Attention and hyperactivity are common in many disorders and, indeed, many more disorders in child psychiatry, and there is clearly poor separation of condition at a clinical level. Measurement issues are common. In relation to comorbidity, there are shared risks factors and one disorder creating an increased risk for another disorder. Neil et al. [35] pointed out that there are correlated liabilities where the risk factors of the two disorders correlate. There are social deficits in both ADHD and autism with overlap from an etiological point of view, but with ADHD the social deficits are more impulsive, and with autism, the social deficits can again be impulsive, but also, they can be due to lack of social know-how and theory of mind deficits. There is no sharp division here.

In a study of ADHD combined type, with one or more siblings, the diagnosis of autism was excluded at the beginning, and siblings with ADHD were compared with siblings without ADHD by Mulligan et al. [36]. They wrote that phenotypic correlation of ADHD and autism symptoms was 0.71 and that 32% of this correlation was due to shared familial characteristics but with a higher percentage for male ADHD probands. There was a trend for children with high ADHD symptoms to have high autism symptoms, as measured by the Social Communication Questionnaire. ADHD probands with definite language disorder or motor disorder had significantly higher symptoms of autism than those without. This study showed that autism symptoms as part of the ADHD phenotype were partly true. These were familial. Probands with autistic traits tend to have siblings with autistic traits, and probands without autistic traits tend to have affected siblings without autistic traits. Finally, latent class analysis of SCQ symptoms in probands with ADHD combined type showed the following clusters of autism symptoms: 31% with few or no symptoms of autism, 22.5% with repetitive and stereotyped behaviour, 21% with communication domain symptoms, 18.5% communication and reciprocal interaction domains and 7% who had symptoms in all three domains.

The percentage of phenotypic correlation due to shared familial influences (autistic symptoms and ADHD) was 35% for the whole group and 62% for males and 12% for females. In a family with a male child with ADHD and comorbid autistic symptoms, a second child with ADHD is also likely to have comorbid autistic symptoms (not so female), which suggest a different aetiology according to sex. Gillberg's [37] disorder of attention, motor control and perception would be showing similar findings. Fifty percent of children with DAMP had autistic features.

Children with oppositional defiant disorder and conduct disorder have more autistic traits than children without these comorbid disorders and ADHD [38]. Children with ADHD have more subthreshold symptoms of autism. Children with combined ADHD and social communication deficits are at increased risk of motor and language disorders. Overall, this shows the massive heterogeneity that is evident in child psychiatry classifications, and clearly, ADHD is not a homogenous disorder. Forty two percent of children with ADHD had few symptoms of autism. That autism symptoms are part of the ADHD phenotype is partly true. Autistic traits in ADHD are familial. This again supports the lack of a sharp overlap between neurodevelopmental disorders, here, autism and ADHD.

8. Personal classification system

If I was to plan an assessment programme in child psychiatry again from the start, I would assess the following dimensions: social reciprocity, pragmatic language, oppositionality, working memory, delinquency, attention, impulsivity, activity, capacity to read non-verbal behaviour, preservation of sameness and fixations.

This would be a transdiagnostic approach.

9. Personality disorder as a developmental disorder

A not insignificant number of personality disorders are developmental disorders. This will require further research. One example is schizoid personality disorder. Another is paranoid personality disorder and, another, borderline personality disorder. Obsessive compulsive personality disorder could be also included in this group. There's quite a good case for narcissistic personality disorder to be included. An older term, anankastic personality disorder [39], could also be included. Many individuals with psychopathy have a developmental disorder, and a group of these have been called criminal autistic psychopathy [40]. There is a clear overlap between psychopathy and autism spectrum disorders. This is despite some research showing that persons with psychopathy have good theory of mind skills, while persons with autism don't. Nevertheless, more recent research has shown that particularly persons with high IQ can have good theory of mind skills while, at the same time, having autism.

10. Cognitive empathy and theory of mind: automatic perspective taking

Blair [41] stated that "cognitive empathy or theory of mind is intact in individuals with psychopathy". These ideas have been very seriously undermined by Drayton et al. [42] in relation to automatic perspective taking. Previous research did not take the complexity of cognitive empathy into account, and this led to serious misunderstandings of cognitive empathy. Drayton et al. [42] point out that "automatic theory of mind processes are engaged when an individual unintentionally represents the perspective of another person," also called "altercentric interference". Drayton et al. [42] suggest that "psychopathic individuals have a diminished propensity to automatically think from another's perspective, which may be the cognitive root of their deficits in social functioning and moral behaviour". Drayton et al. [42] raise, for this author, the possible failure of previous research on theory of mind and psychopathy, failing "to tap into a critical component of normal theory of mind processing; or tendency to take other's perspective automatically". Drayton et al. [42] defined "automatic theory of mind processes" as an individual representing "the thoughts and feelings of another person without intending to do so". They also point out that psychopathic individuals have a previously unobserved cognitive deficit that might explain their patterns of destructive and anti-social behaviour, that is, ... failure "to automatically take the perspective of others, but can deliberately (controlled), take the perspective of others". These findings suggest that psychopathic individuals have the ability to take the perspective of others but lack the propensity to do so. It seems they can pass theory of mind tasks in the research situation but fail to do so in the real world situation. This is one of the endless problems of laboratory research not translating into the "real world," that is, the clinical world. This lack of generalisation can be a serious flaw in academic psychological research. Drayton et al. [42] note that "psychopathic individuals do show deficits in their ability to understand what others are feeling but this capacity to represent other feelings appears to be distinct from capacity to represent what others see and believe". They also point out that "psychopathic individuals appear to represent other's perspective in a relatively typical manner when doing so. It is goal-conducive and yet is able to ignore other's perspective when it is not conducive". This means that all previous theory of mind research on psychopathy missed the fundamental point of the deficit of automatic perspective of others. Drayton et al. [42] point out that "this combination of relatively intact deliberative Theory of Mind but impaired spontaneous theory of mind may allow psychopathic individuals to use information about others' mental states to achieve their own ends, while at the same avoid the, 'cost,' of automatically representing other's mental states, resulting in callous and chronic criminal behaviour". They have no empathic interest in other minds, except getting their own egocentric desires met.

In relation to psychiatry, there's a sharp difference between findings in university laboratories and the findings in clinical practice. Research groups are very rarefied and very often do not represent what is found in the general population, clinically. An example is autism defined by the Autism Diagnostic Interview or Autism Diagnostic Observational Scale which give you a very narrow definition of autism, very unlike what you find in the general population which is the broader autism phenotype [43].

Asperger originally defined persons with autism as being autistic psychopaths, which Frith [44] described as autistic psychopathy or autistic personality disorder. In actual fact, there is a lot of truth in Asperger's [27] definition of autistic psychopaths. This has been brought back now with the terms criminal autistic psychopathy [40, 45]. Indeed, the following could be seen as synonyms, autistic psychopathy, autistic personality disorder, high-functioning autism and Asperger's syndrome.

The kind of criminality seen in autism (criminal autistic psychopathy) would include arson, stalking, sex offences and strange repetitive crimes. According to the Centers for Disease Control [30], developmental disorders are characterised by problems with language, mobility, self-help and independent living. There is a myth that ASD and personality disorder and psychopathy are completely different. There is also a myth that autism and Asperger's syndrome have little or no relationship with criminality and serious murder. Patricia Howlin [46] stated "little, if any significant association between autism and criminal offending". This is clearly not supported by my reading of the literature [40]. Sipponma [47] pointed out that 27% of adult offenders in her study met criteria for autism spectrum disorder. These could be called criminal autistic psychopathy. Ashead and Sarkar [48] described correctly personality disorders as "developmental in nature", and they noted that personality regulates social relationships, arousal impulsivity and emotions, as well as self-directedness and self-soothing as well as verbal and non-verbal communication problems. What is of interest is that all of these areas are abnormal in ASD and personality disorder.

Ashead and Sarkar [48] note the following clusters of personality disorders: odd, eccentric behaviour; anti-social, borderline and narcissistic personality disorders; fearful and anxious behaviour; and avoidant, dependent and obsessive compulsive.

All these clusters, clearly at a descriptive level, overlap with ASD. Ashead and Sarkar [48] describe the following features of personality disorder:

- Emotional indifference
- Anger, suspicion and fearfulness
- Fears of others attacking and threatening them
- Brief psychotic episodes

- Odd beliefs
- Magical thinking
- Preoccupation and ruminations
- Identity confusion
- Empathy problems
- Major problems in in-patient units
- Failure to confirm to social norms
- Social relationship problems
- Social reciprocity problems
- Impulsivity
- Irrationality
- Disregard for safety of self and others
- Reduced reaction to upset in other people
- Preoccupation with one or more stereotyped patterns of behaviour
- Problems with emotional processing
- Emotional detection problems
- Reduced observing self
- Reduced self-awareness and capacity to decentre the self
- Egocentricity
- Low affiliation and harm avoidance

All of these features also occur in autism spectrum disorders. Of course, in a way, this is not surprising since the boundaries between most psychiatric disorders are fluid and we do not have an accurate, categorical diagnosis at this point in time, assuming we ever will.

It's interesting that Wolfe [49], in her group of schizoid disorder overlapping with Asperger's syndrome, found "fraudulent behaviour and pathological lying"; in that, 5 out of 13 had "falsely reported their parents of being cruel to them" and "had used aliases".

There is a myth that persons with high-functioning autism cannot lie. This is utterly false, as from a clinical perspective, many parents complain to me about their children with high-functioning autism being what they call "inveterate liars". Of course, the great majority of persons with autism are the opposite and are incredibly honest, open, moral, etc. These features of autism spectrum disorder occur in the general population, as do features of personality disorder. It's only when you get to a certain threshold that you would get a diagnosis of autism or personality disorder. In truth, we need a new classification system in psychiatry again. The problem is that most of our current disorders overlap and are therefore not independent. We need to go back from a classificatory point of view, to a pre-Kraepelin period and, in a way, that is, what the NIMH is stating with their transdiagnostic research.

There are a number of phrases associated with personality disorder, which could also be associated with autism spectrum disorder:

i. Schizoid personality, “you can knock, but nobody’s home” [50].

ii. Schizotypal personality, “I’m eccentric, different, strange” [50].

iii. Paranoid personality, “you can’t trust anybody” [50].

iv. Borderline personality, “I will be very angry, if you try to leave me” [50].

v. The sadistic personality, “I will savour your suffering” [50]. This particularly refers to criminal autistic psychopathy and serial killers.

vi. Narcissistic personality, “my command is your wish” [50].

11. Conclusion

The future of psychiatry will be neurodevelopmental. Psychiatrists will focus on these conditions. Mild psychiatric conditions will be dealt with by psychiatric counsellors and psychologists, using psychotherapeutic interventions. This will allow psychiatrists to become neuropsychiatrists which they are all already moving towards. The “blaming” culture of attributing these disorders to mothers’ inadequacies will then be at an end. The neurodevelopmental spectrum is far wider and far more important than suggested by DSM 5 [2, 3].

Author details

Michael Fitzgerald*
Department of Psychiatry, Trinity College, Dublin, Ireland

*Address all correspondence to: sarahwin@connect.hku.hk

References

[1] Bowlby J. Attachment and Loss. Vol. 2. Harmondsworth: Penguin Books; 1981

[2] American Psychiatric Association. DSM 5. Washington DC: APA; 2013

[3] Mazefsky C, White S. Adults with autism. In: Volkmar F, Rogers S, Paul R, Pelphrey K, editors. Handbook of Autism and Pervasive Developmental Disorders. New Jersey: Wiley; 2014

[4] Lord C, Rutter M, Dilavore P, Risi S. Autistic Diagnostic Observation Schedule. Los Angeles, CA: Western Psychological Services; 2002

[5] Evans B. How autism became autism. History of Human Sciences. July 2013;**26**(3):3-31

[6] Fitzgerald M. Overlap between autism and schizophrenia: History and current status. Advances in Mental Health and Intellectual Disabilities. 2014;**8**:1-8

[7] Kolvin I. Studies in childhood psychosis 1. Diagnostic criteria and classification. British Journal of Psychiatry. 1971;**118**:381-384

[8] Sullivan P, Magnussen C, Boman M, et al. Family history of schizophrenia and bipolar disorder as a risk factor for autism. Archives of General Psychiatry. 2012;**69**(11):1099-1103

[9] Scull A. Madness and Civilisation. London: Thames & Hudson; 2015

[10] Rutter M. Classification and categorisation in child psychiatry. Journal of Child Psychology and Psychiatry. 1965;**6**(71):81

[11] Rutter M. Concepts of autism: A review of research. Journal of Child Psychology and Child Psychiatry. 1968;**9**:1-25

[12] Abel K. The Holy Grail of schizophrenia research: Are we closer to understanding its causes and preventing new cases? Irish Psychiatrists. 2011;**12**(4):112-114

[13] Rapaport J, Chavez A, Greenstein D, Addington A, Gogtay N. Autism Spectrum disorders and childhood onset schizophrenia: Clinical and biological contributions to our relationship revisited. Journal of the American Academy of Child & Adolescent Psychiatry. 2009;**48**(1):10-18

[14] Carroll L, Owen M. Genetic overlap between autism, schizophrenia and bipolar disorder. Genome Medicine. 30 October 2009;**1**(10):102

[15] Fatemi SH. The role of Reelin in autism. In: Hollander E, Kolevzon A, Coyle JT, editors. Textbook of Autism Spectrum Disorders. Washington, DC: American Psychiatric Publishing; 2011

[16] Burbach JP, Van Der Zwaag B. Contact in the genetics of autism and schizophrenia. Trends in Neurosciences. 2009;**32**(2):69-72

[17] Rutter M. Psychiatric disorders in early childhood. In: Coppen A, Walk A, editors. Recent Developments in Schizophrenia: A Symposium. London: RMPA; 1967

[18] Stone W, Iguchi L. Do apparent overlaps between schizophrenia and autism spectrum disorders reflect superficial similarities or etiological commonalities? North American Journal of Medicine and Science. 2011;**4**(3):124-133

[19] Solomon M, Olsen E, Niendam T, Carter C. From lumping to splitting and back again. Schizophrenia Research. 2011;**131**(1-3):146-151

[20] Frith C. Cognitive Neuropsychology of Schizophenia. Earlbaum: Hove Germany; 1992

[21] Craddock N, Owen MJ. The Kraepelian dichotomy: Going, going... but still not gone. The British Journal of Psychiatry. 2010;**196**:92-95

[22] Sporn AL. Pervasive developmental disorder and childhood onset schizophrenia: Co-morbid disorder or phenotypic variant of a very early onset illness. Biological Psychiatry. 2004;**55**(10):989-994

[23] Rutter M. Prognosis: Psychotic children in adolescence and early adult life. In: Wing JK, editor. Childhood Autism: Clinical, Educational and Social Aspects. London: Pergamon Press; 1966

[24] Kolb L. Noyes Modern Clinical Psychiatry. Philadelphia: Saunders; 1968

[25] WHO. International Classification of Mental and Behavioural Disorder. ICD 10. Geneva: WHO; 1973

[26] Kanner L. Problems in the nosology and psychodynamics of early infantile autism. American Journal of Orthopsychiatry. 1949;**19**(3):416-426

[27] Asperger H. Die, "Autistischen Psychopathen". In: Kindesalter. Archive fur Psychiatrie und Nervenkrankheiten. 1944;**117**:76-136

[28] Gillberg C, Schumann H. Social class and infantile autism. Journal of Autism and Developmental Disorders. 1982;**12**(3):223-228

[29] Baird G, Simonoff E, Pickles A, Chandler Charman T. The prevalence of disorders of autism spectrum disorder in a population cohort of children in South Thames: The special needs and autism project. Lancet. 2006;**268**:210-215

[30] CDC. Autism. Atlanta: Centre for Disease Control; 2018/2012

[31] Canitano R, Vivanti G. Tics and Tourette's syndrome in autism. Autism. 2007;**11**(1):19-28

[32] Stein DJ. Neurobiology of obsessive-compulsive spectrum disorders. Biological Psychiatry. 2000;**47**(4):296-304

[33] Meir SM, Petersen L, Mors O, et al. Obsessive-compulsive disorder and autism spectrum disorder: Longitudinal and off-spring risk. PLoS One. 2015;**10**(11):eo141703. DOI: 10:1371/Journal.pone014703.eCollection 2015

[34] Caron C, Rutter M. Co-morbidity in child psychopathy. Journal of Child Psychology and Psychiatry. 1991;**32**:1063-1080

[35] Neale MC, Kendler KS. Models of co-morbidity for multifactorial disorder. American Journal of Human Genetics. 1995;**57**:935-953

[36] Mulligan A. Symptoms of Autism and ADHD: A Familial Trait. Saarbrucken: Lambert; 2009

[37] Gillberg C. Deficits in attention, motor control and perception. Archives of Disease in Childhood. 2003;**88**:904-910

[38] Mulligan A, Anney R, Fitzgerald M, Steinhausen HC, Rotherberger A, Minderaa R, et al. Autistic symptoms in ADHD: A familial trait with correlates with conduct, oppositional defiant, language and motor disorders. Journal of Autism and Developmental Disorders. 2008. DOI: 1001/S10803-008-0621-3

[39] Fitzgerald M. Missed diagnosis of Aspergers syndrome as Anankastic personality disorder. Autism. 2002;**6**(4):435

[40] Fitzgerald M. Young, Violent and Dangerous to Know. New York: Nova Science; 2010

[41] Blair J. Psychopathy: Cognitive and neural dysfunction. 2013;**15**(2):181-190

[42] Drayton L, Santos R. Psychopaths fail automatically to take the perspectives of others. 2018. DOI: 10.1073/pnas.1721903115

[43] Baird G, Simonoff E, Pickles A, Chandler Charman T. The prevalence of disorders of autism spectrum disorder in a population cohort of children in South Thames: The Special Needs and Autism Project. Lancet. 2006;**268**:210-215

[44] Frith U. Autism and Aspergers Syndrome. Cambridge: Cambridge University Press; 1991

[45] Fitzgerald M. Young, violent and dangerous to know. New York: Nova Science; 2010

[46] Howlin P. Autism preparing for adulthood. London: Rutledge; 1997

[47] Siponmma L, Jonson C, Nyden A, Gillberg C. Juvenile and young adult mentally disordered offenders: The role of neuropsychiatric disorders. Journal of American Academy of Psychiatry and Law. 2001;**29**:420-426

[48] Ashead G, Sarkar J. The nature of personality disorder. Advances in Psychiatric Treatment. May. 2012:162-172

[49] Wolf S. The Life Path of Unusual Children. London: Rutledge; 1995

[50] Millon T, Davis R, Millon C. Personality Disorder in Modern Life. New York: Wiley; 2000

Section 2

Autism and Schizophrenia

Chapter 2

Autism: A Neurodevelopmental Disorder and a Stratum for Comorbidities

Marwa Mahmoud Saleh and Aya Adel

Abstract

Autism is a neurodevelopmental disorder which is more common in males than females. It is characterized by social communication disorders and restricted repetitive behaviors. There is wide heterogeneity in its etiology, clinical presentations, management and consequently prognosis. Although the etiology of autism remains unclear, the most currently proven theory is that it is a complex neurodevelopmental disorder that displays "brain network abnormalities". fMRI studies have shown decreased brain connectivity or functional synchronization between frontal and more posterior cortical regions. Dynamic brain activity through high resolution electroencephalograghy (EEG) has revealed local overconnectivity and long-range underconnectivity. This disrupted connectivity pattern would involve connectivity between hemispheres (corpus callosum), together with axonal and synaptic connectivity within each hemisphere. Inconsistent morphometric changes involving both gray and white matter structure also exist. Clinically, autism is associated with multiple comorbidities (somatic, neurologic and psychiatric); some of which are attention deficit hyperactivity disorder, dyspraxia, and sensory processing disorders.

Keywords: autism, MRI findings, comorbidities

1. Introduction

According to the American Psychiatric Association's Diagnostic and Statistical Manual of Mental Disorders (DSM-5), autism spectrum disorders (ASDs) are characterized by social communication impairment and repetitive restricted behaviors. Autism is the commonest neurodevelopmental disorder in the scope of ASD. The social impairment affects both verbal and nonverbal communication [1].

1.1 Social deficits

There is lack of social attention and attention shifting in the autistic children in parallel with lack of development of joint attention skills [2]. The affected children display emotional reactions that do not associate with the surrounding events. They show negative emotions more frequently than positive emotions, without justifiable cause for inducing either response. Their play patterns are solitary, and they do not develop typical interactive social play with other children [3].

Abnormality in face perception is a core feature in autism. Face processing includes unchangeable facial features as those relating to gender and identity and changeable facial features such as emotional expression and gaze direction. Autistic children ignore looking at faces of others and are unable to understand facial expressions. Fixation time on the eye area of the face is reduced in ASD individuals. Opposite to what occurs in typically developing individuals, processing of gaze direction in autism experimentally produced more activation in fusiform gyrus for averted than for direct look. This was termed "covert attention," as autistic individuals are visually attentive and perceptive, but in an atypical manner.

During recognition of neutral faces, the autistic children exhibit a reduced activation of fusiform gyrus, superior temporal sulcus, amygdala, and occipital lobes, the primary areas for face recognition. In spite of this fact, autistic children showed typical activation when looking at familiar faces like that of a mother. Inferior temporal, middle, and inferior frontal gyri are also involved in face processing. It is important to note that reduced connectivity in brain networks between areas of face processing emerged as a holistic approach to explain the atypical face perception in autistic children [4].

The social processing involves social cognition and social motivation. Social cognition involves processes like attention, memory, and theory of mind, by which the person infers the internal state of others. Social motivation resembles directing attention to socially relevant stimuli and enjoying social activities. Both activities depend on the function of face processing. So it is related to the areas of face processing in addition to striatum (social interaction) and orbitofrontal cortex (social motivation) [5]. Impaired connectivity in social executive functions is present in ASD children [6].

1.2 Restricted repetitive behavior

Autistic individuals resist change in their daily routine or the familiar surroundings. They do not explore while playing, and the toys are manipulated with little creativity or symbolic function. They are cognitively inflexible, as they may be preoccupied with parts of objects, or attached to unusual objects or movements, as watching the rotatory activity of fans. They could show stereotypic repetitive behavior that may be injurious to self or others. They tend to have a repetitive sensory motor behavior, insistence on sameness, and sometimes self-injurious acts [7].

2. Body

2.1 Etiologies

Autism has a strong complex genetic basis. Abnormalities in gene expression affect the molecular, synaptic, cellular, and brain network levels. There is variability in results of brain imaging studies [magnetic resonance imaging (MRI) and diffusion tensor imaging (DTI)] in autism, which report structural cerebral changes and functional connectivity disruptions. Alterations in overall gray and white matter volume and in regional lobes and gyri were witnessed.

Early brain overgrowth, especially in an early age of 2–3 years old toddlers remains, however, one of the most replicated findings. Compared with typically developing children, global gray matter (GM) and white matter (WM) volumes were significantly increased and also right superior temporal gyrus regional GM and WM volumes. Higher fractional anisotropy value was also observed in the corpus callosum, posterior cingulate cortex, and limbic lobes of autistic children

[8]. The converging findings of structural and white matter abnormalities in autism suggest that alterations in neural anatomy of different brain regions may be involved in the associated behavioral and cognitive deficits in this disorder.

Nevertheless, recent neural models of autism spectrum disorders have moved the focus from a lesion model to connectivity disorder model. Aberrant conductivity between different brain regions in autism is currently the most frequently addressed neurodevelopmental model. Minshew and Williams [9] have implicated intra-hemispheric connectivity to be mainly involved in the disorder. Vissers et al. [10] have studied functional and structural brain connectivity in individuals with high functioning individuals with ASD. They supported the findings that long-range cortico-cortical functional and structural pathways displayed weaker connectivity in people with ASD than in controls, but with less evidence for local overconnectivity. Other researchers have supported a local overconnectivity and long-range underconnectivity pattern of brain functioning in autism through the use of high-resolution electroencephalography (EEG) [11]. Cortical underconnectivity between brain regions, especially the frontal cortex and more posterior areas, is relatively well established in autism. This supports the view that there is weaker coordination between different parts of the brain that should be working together to accomplish complex social and language tasks. This is opposite to what is occurring during normal development [12].

In this cerebral connectivity disorder of autism, the cerebellum has also been strongly implicated. Although the role of cerebellum as error detector and coordinator of movement and balance was the typical portrait of cerebellar function, yet recognition of nonmotor functions of the cerebellum has recently come into view. While some parts of the cerebellum are predominantly connected to sensorimotor cortex, other connections project to cognitive and affective regions and comprise a large fraction of cerebellar connectivity [13]. Impairment of these connections was also reported in autism.

As a model for aberrant conductivity in autism, we could consider the reported comments about deviations in corpus callosum, white matter, and neurotransmitters. So, brain connectivity includes connectivity between the two hemispheres done mainly by the corpus callosum (CC), or between multiple areas in the brain accomplished by tracts in white matter and by synapses and neurotransmitters. People need this connectivity as different regions of the brain need to communicate in order to identify a face, understand, and respond to others and to different social situations. Disruption of white matter tracts in regions related to social functioning is implicated in autism [14]. In autism, defective joint attention was related to decreased connectivity and synchronization between posterior involuntary attention related to responding to joint attention (RJA) and anterior volitional joint attention related to initiating joint attention (IJA) [15].

The corpus callosum (CC) constitutes the main commissural tract between the two hemispheres (more than 200 million axons). A study by Hardan et al. [16] that investigated the corpus callosum by MRI-based morphometry has identified decreased total volume of CC and several of its seven subdivisions. This was found in other studies and could reflect in the form of social deficits, repetitive behavior, and sensory processing abnormalities.

There are neural circuits for social cognition, which involves attention, memory, motivation, and emotion. Abnormalities in social brain structures and circuitry that are modulated by several neurotransmitters and neuromodulators have been linked, through human fMRI and animal research, to disorders of social functioning as in autism [17]. Neurotransmitter systems involved in autism spectrum disorders have been identified as GABA, glutamate, serotonin, catecholamines, and acetyl choline [18, 19].

In the area of communication abilities, the gifts of memory, understanding, emotional expression, and learning are used on a daily basis. Sometimes, these abilities are disrupted due to deviant central nervous system development (neurodevelopmental disease), which includes long-range underconnectivity and local overconnectivity. Conditions like autism spectrum disorders (ASDs), and attention-deficit hyperactivity disorder (ADHD), can emerge secondary to these disruptions.

2.2 Comorbidities

Autism is in comorbidity relationship with many disorders as epilepsy [20], with intellectual disability and with attention deficit hyperactivity disorder (ADHD) [21]. Other disorders such as fragile X, Rett syndrome, and tuberous sclerosis are also described. Intellectual disability, epilepsy, and ADHD can share a common neurobiological basis and are factors of poor prognosis of autism [22]. Comorbidities are the main reasons for referral to outpatient clinics and admission to hospitals. Among the most challenging co-existing dysfunctions are cognitive impairment, hyperactivity, sensory processing disorders, and dyspraxia. They mask and hinder proper diagnosis and are the cause of inadequate management [23, 24]. That is why Gadow et al. [25] strongly recommend looking at the presence of comorbidities before starting any treatment for autism.

Among the several comorbidities associated with autism, this chapter is going to focus on three commonly encountered conditions: ADHD, dyspraxia, and sensory processing disorders. ADHD, characterized by symptoms of inattention and hyperactivity/impulsivity [1], is frequently associated with autism. The diagnosis of this disorder is difficult to make when present concomitant with autism. In fact, in previous versions of DSM, ASD and ADHD were regarded as distinct disorders. The child was either diagnosed as ASD or ADHD, with a common negative impact mainly on semantics and pragmatics in both of their language profiles. A diagnosis of ASD was considered an exclusion criterion for the diagnosis of ADHD. However, recent research recognizes considerable clinical, genetic, and neuropsychological overlap between ASD and ADHD and within the DSM-5, and ADHD can now be diagnosed in conjunction with ASD.

Both disorders share a portion of their heritable etiology. About 50–72% of the contributing genetic factors overlap between ASD and ADHD. Furthermore, similar deficits in executive function, social cognition, and motor speed have been linked to both ASD and ADHD [26]. Both diseases have similar neuropathology and also share similar symptomatology with considerable overlap in their core and associated symptoms and a frequent overlap in their comorbid conditions. Consequently, it is apparent that ASD and ADHD diagnoses belong to a broader spectrum of neurodevelopmental disorders, an abnormal connectivity spectrum disorder, which results from neural long-range underconnectivity and short-range overconnectivity. Many psychopathological, neuropsychological, brain imaging, genetic, and medical findings have suggested that these disorders are part of a continuum [27].

There are some recorded similarities between these two disorders. First, males are more commonly affected as having ASD or ADHD than females. A review of automated medical records of children revealed the percentages of males evaluated in ASD and ADHD groups were 80.4 and 77.7%, respectively [28]. Second, both disorders are often diagnosed later during childhood. The respective median ages for a diagnosis of ASD or ADHD were 4.7 and 6.4 years [29]. Third, these disorders share symptomatology, showing considerable overlap in the core and associated symptoms, that is, issues with attention, impulsivity, repetitive behaviors, impairments in socialization and communication, anxiety, sensory processing abnormalities, and ritualistic behaviors, such as counting, ordering, repeating or arranging [30]. Fourth, these disorders share neuropathology.

In clinical practice, the often reported co-occurrence of ASD and ADHD might link them in several pathways: inattention/impulsivity and social ineptness; hyperactivity and stereotypic, repetitive behaviors; and the semantic pragmatic language deficit. The clinical links between ASD and ADHD are variable and strong, as well as the neurodevelopmental basis [31].

Another comorbid disorder that occurs frequently with autism is dyspraxia. Praxis is the ability to conceptualize, plan, and successfully complete motor actions in novel situations. It is a naturally emerging skill that develops as the child interacts successfully with people and objects in the environment and enables the child to learn new skills by watching, imitating, and exploring.

Developmental dyspraxia is the failure to acquire the ability to perform appropriate complex motor actions. It is related to problems of transitive gestures (pantomimed tool use), intransitive actions (symbolic gestures such as waving goodbye), imitative actions (such as imitating meaningless hand or body postures), motor planning, and difficulty conceptualizing novel ways to interact with objects [32]. Many researches have illustrated that children with autism have difficulties in all categorizations of developmental dyspraxia [33].

Autistic children have impaired motor function, including clumsy gait, impairments in coordination, balance, and posture, and abnormal performance of skilled gestures [34]. The deficient performance of skilled motor gestures secondary to command, imitation, or tool use is actually one of the most consistent motor signs in autism [35], which is also consistent with "developmental dyspraxia" [36].

Motor praxis concerns have been reported for children with ASD based on scores from a variety of motor tests and movement observations. Autistic children have been reported to show deficits in their ability to produce meaningful and meaningless gestures on command, imitate demonstrated gestures without objects, and imitate gestures involving real or imaginary tool use. These praxis abilities require the child to interpret sensory information and then formulate internal action models. That is why some researchers suggested that impairments in dyspraxia may contribute to the primary features of the disorder, including impaired social interaction and communication skills [37].

Besides motor praxis dysfunction, speech-language pathologists have observed co-occurrence of childhood apraxia of speech (CAS) with autism. CAS is difficulty in coordinating volitional motor movements that are required for clear and intelligible speech. It can be witnessed in verbal and nonverbal autistic children in the form of defective vowel production, prosody, and difficulty in imitation of speech sounds. This definitely augments the problem of social and language delay in autism and presents a big obstacle in the pathway of verbal language. The possible presence of this obstacle might to be considered and evaluated before the start of therapy because comorbidity between autism and CAS is still vague, and verbal language remains the ultimate goal of success of therapy from the parents' perspective.

A recent research, however, has found autism and apraxia of speech to be highly comorbid. A 3-year study on 30 children with communication delay has shown that 63.6% of children originally diagnosed as having autism had speech apraxia and 36.8% of children originally diagnosed with speech apraxia had autism. The drawn conclusion from this study was that two-thirds of the children initially diagnosed with autism also had apraxia [38]. It is advisable that children with autism are observed for signs of apraxia and children with apraxia are observed for signs of autism. This observation in clinical practice translates to the fact that language delay in autistic children may not be purely of an "autistic" origin.

A third comorbidity commonly occurring with autism is sensory processing disorders (SPDs). Sensory processing means the brain's ability to register, organize, and make sense of the information received through one's senses. SPDs are commonly encountered with autism and have recently been included among the diagnostic criteria in DSM-5. They might even be encountered in children with other developmental disabilities and in typically developing children as well. When sensory processing is dysfunctional, the individual's ability to cope with the demands of the environment would be disrupted [39].

Suarez [39] have drawn a hierarchical classification of SPD, dividing it into three main categories: sensory-based motor disorder (poor motor planning and/or postural instability resulting from improper processing of information from the senses), sensory discrimination disorder (inability to perceive differences and similarities in data received from the senses which can make reading very challenging), and sensory modulation disorder (impairment in intensity and nature of behavior in response to sensory information). The latter subtype is the one commonly encountered in autism, and it has three subcategories: sensory hyperresponsiveness, sensory hyporesponsiveness, and sensory seeking.

Consequently, autistic individuals with SPD can be categorized into hyporesponsive, hyperresponsive, or sensory seekers. The hyperresponsiveness means overreaction to sensations that are typically harmless or not even perceived by others. Inappropriate behavior outbursts may be triggered by feeling textures on the skin (clothes and food), movement activities (swinging), or hearing sudden noises (doorbells). They are overcautious and resist changes in daily routine. The hyporesponsiveness requires intense sensory input to attract the attention of the child as sustained loud sound. Symptoms include not responding to name, or even to painful stimuli. Sensory seeking is characterized by excessive drive for certain sensory stimuli, as putting things in the mouth or touching people to the point of annoying them. Sensory seeking may be injurious or disrupting to the development of meaningful social relationships.

The proposed division of sensory modulation disorder into distinct subcategories serves theoretical understanding of the problem. Clinically, however, the autistic children show a mixture of symptoms that belong to more than one subcategory. They might be annoyed by ordinary sounds to the degree that they cover their ears, and they might be attracted to very fine sounds as the sound of turning of a page, or they might ignore a very loud sound [40]. Some researchers have reported positive associations between hyporeactivity and social communication symptom severity, whereas others have found that child hyperreactivity is likely to negatively affect family life and social adaptive behaviors of school-age children [41].

Questions have arisen regarding the relation of restricted repetitive behavior and sensory processing disorders (SPDs) in autism. Gabriels et al. [42] have suggested the presence of a subgroup with frequent restricted repetitive behavior and multiple abnormal sensory responses due to significant relationship between both. Hyper- or hyporeactivity to sensory stimuli have actually been included in DSM-5 as one of the forms that exist under the title of "Restricted Repetitive patterns of Behavior."

3. Conclusion

Autism is a diverse manifold neurodevelopmental disorder affecting many of the child's abilities. Some disabilities are core features, while others are comorbidities. The clinical picture therefore differs from one child to another. The main deficit in neurodevelopment is that of aberrant connectivity.

Author details

Marwa Mahmoud Saleh* and Aya Adel
Phoniatric Unit, Department of Otolaryngology, Ain Shams University, Cairo, Egypt

*Address all correspondence to: marwa.saleh7@gmail.com

References

[1] American Psychiatric Association. Diagnostic and Statistical Manual of Mental Disorders. 5th ed. Arlington, VA: American Psychiatric Publishing; 2013

[2] Saleh M, Adel A. Joint attention impairment in autism: Clinical picture, rationale and functional MRI findings. In: Fitzgerald M, Yip J, editors. Autism. Rijeka, Crotia: IntechOpen; 2017. DOI: 10.5772/65662. Available from: https://www.intechopen.com/books/autism-paradigms-recent-research-and-clinical-applications/joint-attention-impairment-in-autism-clinical-picture-rationale-and-functional-mri-findings

[3] Hutman T, Chela MK, Gillespie-Lynch K, Sigman M. Selective visual attention at twelve months: Signs of autism in early social interactions. Journal of Autism and Developmental Disorders. 2011;**13**(1):512-516. DOI: 10.1007/s10803-011-1262-5

[4] Nomi JS, Uddin LQ. Face processing in autism spectrum disorders: From brain regions to brain networks. Neuropsychologia. 2015;**71**:201-216. DOI: 10.1016/j.neuropsychologia.2015.03.029

[5] Hutchins TL, Prelock PA, Bonazinga L. Psychometric evaluation of the theory of mind inventory (TOMI): A study of typically developing children and children with autism spectrum disorder. Journal of Autism and Developmental Disorders. 2012;**42**(3):327-341. DOI: 10.1007/s10803-011-1244-7

[6] Bernas A, Aldenkamp AP, Zinger S. Wavelet coherence-based classifier: A resting-state functional MRI study on neurodynamics in adolescents with high-functioning autism. Computer Methods and Programs in Biomedicine. 2018;**154**:143-151. DOI: 10.1016/j.cmpb.2017.11.017

[7] Kim SH, Lord C. Restricted and repetitive behaviors in toddlers and preschoolers with autism spectrum disorders based on the autism diagnostic observation schedule (ADOS). Autism Research. 2010;**3**(4):162-173. DOI: 10.1002/aur.142

[8] Xiao Z, Qiu T, Ke X, Xiao X, Xiao T, Liang F, et al. Autism spectrum disorder as early neurodevelopmental disorder: Evidence from the brain imaging abnormalities in 2-3 years old toddlers. Journal of Autism and Developmental Disorders. 2014;**44**(7):1633-1640. DOI: 10.1007/s10803-014-2033-x

[9] Minshew NJ, Williams DL. The new neurobiology of autism: Cortex, connectivity and neuronal organization. Archives of Neurology. 2007;**6**:945-950. DOI: 10.1001/archneur.64.7.945

[10] Vissers ME, Cohen MX, Geurts HM. Brain connectivity and high functioning autism: A promising path of research that needs refined models, methodological convergence, and stronger behavioral links. Neuroscience and Biobehavioral Reviews. 2012;**36**:604-625. DOI: 10.1016/j.neubiorev.2011.09.003

[11] Barttfeld P, Wicker B, Cukier S, Navarta S, Lew S, Sigman M. A big-world network in ASD: Dynamical connectivity analysis reflects a deficit in long-range connections and an excess of short-range connections. Neuropsychologia. 2011;**49**:254-263. DOI: 10.1016/j.neuropsychologia.2010.11.024

[12] Kana RK, Murdaugh DL, Libero LE, Pennick MR, Wadsworth HM, Deshpande R, et al. Probing the brain in autism using FMRI and diffusion tensor imaging. Journal of Visualized Experiments. 2011;**55**:3178. DOI: 10.3791/3178

[13] Strick PL, Dum RP, Fiez JA. Cerebellum and nonmotor function. Annual Review of Neuroscience. 2009;**32**:413-434. DOI: 10.1146/annurev.neuro.31.060407.125606

[14] Barnea-Goraly N, Kwon H, Menon V, Eliez S, Lotspeich L, Reiss AL. White matter structure in autism: Preliminary evidence from diffusion tensor imaging. Biological Psychiatry. 2004;**55**(3):323-326

[15] Mundy P, Card J, Fox N. Fourteen-month cortical activity and different infant joint attention skills. Developmental Psychobiology. 2000;**36**:325-338

[16] Hardan AY, Pabalan M, Gupta N, Bansal R, Melhem NM, Fedorov S, et al. Corpus callosum volume in children with autism. Psychiatry Research: Neuroimaging. 2009;**174**(1):57-61. DOI: 10.1016/j.pscychresns.2009.03.005

[17] Fernández M, Mollinedo-Gajate I, Peñagarikano O. Neural circuits for social cognition: Implications for autism. Neuroscience. 2017;**370**:148-162. DOI: 10.1016/j.neuroscience.2017.07.013

[18] Mohammadi M. Comments on Quaak, et al. The dynamics of autism spectrum disorders: How neurotoxic compounds and neurotransmitters interact. International Journal of Environmental Research and Public Health. 2016;**13**(12):1207. DOI: 10.3390/ijerph13121207

[19] Cetin FH, Tunca H, Guney E, Iseri E. Neurotransmitter systems in autism spectrum disorder. In: Fitzgerald M, editor. Autism Spectrum Disorder. Rijeka, Crotia: IntechOpen; 2015. DOI: 10.5772/59122. Available from: https://www.intechopen.com/books/autism-spectrum-disorder-recent-advances/neurotransmitter-systems-in-autism-spectrum-disorder

[20] Tuchman R, Rapin I. Epilepsy in autism. Lancet Neurology. 2002;**1**(6):352-358

[21] Rommelse NNJ, Geurts HM, Franke B, Buitelaar JK, Hartaman CA. A review on cognitive and brain endophenotypes that may be common in autism spectrum disorder and attention-deficit/hyperactivity disorder facilitate the search for pleitropic genes. Neuroscience and Biobehavioral Reviews. 2011;**35**(6):1363-1396. DOI: 10.1016/j.neubiorev.2011.02.015

[22] Rutter M. Autism research, lesson from the past and prospects for the future. Journal of Autism and Developmental Disorders. 2005;**35**(2):241-257

[23] Mouridsen SE, Brønnum-Hansen H, Rich B, Isager T. Mortality and causes of death in autism spectrum disorders: An update. Autism. 2008;**12**(4):403-414. DOI: 10.1177/1362361308091653

[24] Périsse D, Amiet C, Consoli A, Thorel MV, Gourfinkel-An I, Bodeau N, et al. Risk factors of acute behavioral regression in psychiatrically hospitalized adolescents with autism. Journal of Canadian Academy of Child and Adolescent Psychiatry. 2010;**19**(2):100-108

[25] Gadow KD, Devincent CJ, Schneider J. Predictors of psychiatric symptoms in children with an autism spectrum disorder. Journal of Autism and Developmental Disorders. 2008;**38**(9):1710-1720

[26] Sokolova E, Oerlemans AM, Rommelse NN, Groot P, Hartman CA, Glennon JC, et al. A causal and mediation analysis of the comorbidity between attention deficit hyperactivity disorder (ADHD) and autism spectrum disorder (ASD). Journal of Autism and Developmental Disorders. 2017;**47**(6):1595-1604. DOI: 10.1007/s10803-017-3083-7

[27] Kern JK, Geier DA, Sykes LK, Geier MR, Deth RC. Are ASD and ADHD a continuum? A comparison of pathophysiological similarities between the disorders. Journal of Attention Disorders. 2012;**19**(9):805-827. DOI: 10.1177/1087054712459886

[28] Young HA, Geier DA, Geier MR. Thimerosal exposure in infants and neurodevelopmental disorders: An assessment of computerized medical records in the vaccine safety datalink. Journal of the Neurological Sciences. 2008;**271**:110-118. DOI: 10.1016/j.jns.2008.04.002

[29] Kern JK, Geier DA, King PJ, Sykes LK, Mehta J, Geier MR. Shared connectivity issues, symptoms, and comorbidities in autism spectrum disorder, attention deficit/hyperactivity disorder, and tourette syndrome. Brain Connectivity. 2015;**5**(6):321-325. DOI: 10.1089/brain.2014.0324

[30] Grzadzinski R, Di Martino A, Brady E, Mairena MA, O'Neale M, Petkova E, et al. Examining autistic traits in children with ADHD: Does the autism spectrum extend to ADHD? Journal of Autism and Developmental Disorders. 2011;**41**:1178-1191. DOI: 10.1007/s10803-010-1135-3

[31] Leitner Y. The co-occurrence of autism and attention deficit hyperactivity disorder in children—What do we know? Frontiers in Human Neuroscience. 2014;**8**:268. DOI: 10.3389/fnhum.2014.00268

[32] Bodison SC. Developmental dyspraxia and the play skills of children with autism. The American Journal of Occupational Therapy. 2015;**69**(5):1-6. DOI: 10.5014/ajot.2015.017954

[33] MacNeil LK, Mostofsky SH. Specificity of dyspraxia in children with autism. Neuropsychology. 2012;**26**(20):165-171. DOI: 10.1037/a0026955

[34] Gidley Larson JC, Mostofsky SH. Motor deficits in autism. In: Tuchman R, Rapin I, editors. Autism: A Neurological Disorder of Early Brain Development. London: Mac Keith Press for the International Review of Child Neurology Series; 2006. pp. 231-247

[35] Dowell LR, Mahone EM, Mostofsky SH. Associations of postural knowledge and basic motor skill with dyspraxia in autism: Implication for abnormalities in distributed connectivity and motor learning. Neuropsychology. 2009;**23**(5):563-570. DOI: 10.1037/a0015640

[36] Steinman KJ, Mostofsky SH, Denckla MB. Toward a narrower, more pragmatic view of developmental dyspraxia. Journal of Child Neurology. 2010;**25**(1):71-81. DOI: 10.1177/0883073809342591

[37] Bodison S, Mostofsky S. Motor control and motor learning processes in autism spectrum disorders. In: Volkmar FR, Paul R, Rogers SJ, Pelphrey KA, editors. Handbook of Autism and Pervasive Developmental Disorders: Vol. 2. Assessment, Interventions, and Policy. 4th ed. Hoboken, NJ: Wiley; 2014. pp. 354-377

[38] Tierney C, Mayes S, Lohs S, Black A, Gisin E, Veglia M. How valid is the checklist for autism spectrum disorder when a child has apraxia of speech? Journal of Developmental and Behavioral Pediatrics. 2015;**36**(8):569-574. DOI: 10.1097/DBP.0000000000000189

[39] Suarez MA. Sensory processing in children with autism spectrum disorders and impact on functioning. Pediatric Clinics. 2012;**59**(1):203-214. DOI: 10.1016/j.pcl.2011.10.012

[40] DeBoth KK, Reynolds S. A systematic review of sensory-based autism subtypes. Research in Autism Spectrum Disorder. 2017;**36**:44-56

[41] Ben-Sasson A, Carter AS, Briggs-Gowan MJ. Sensory over-responsivity in elementary school: Prevalence and social-emotional correlates. Journal of Abnormal Child Psychology. 2009;**37**:705-716. DOI: 10.1007/s10802-008-9295-8

[42] Gabriels RL, Agnew JA, Miller LJ, Gralla J, Pan Z, Goldson E, et al. Is there a relationship between restricted repetitive behaviors and interests and abnormal sensory response in children with autism spectrum disorders? Research in Autism Spectrum Disorders. 2008;**2**:660-670

Chapter 3

Schizophrenia: Early Recognition and Prevention

Delia Marina Podea, Romina Teodora Moldovan and Laura Cristina Popa

Abstract

Schizophrenia is a heterogenous disorder presenting as episodes of psychosis against a background of cognitive, social, and functional impairments. Schizophrenia, a multifaceted neuropsychiatric disorder, is affecting approximately 1% of the population worldwide. Its onset is the result of a complex interplay of genetic predisposition and environmental factors. The clinical staging model of psychotic disorders implies that early successful treatment may improve prognosis and prevent progression to more severe stages of disorder. So, prevention and early intervention of schizophrenia are correlated with the prodromal phase, especially with "at risk mental state" (ARMS) and the prediction of their transition to a full-blown psychotic disorder. The psychosis prodrome includes nonspecific signs and symptoms (such as depressed mood, anxiety, sleep disturbance, and deterioration in role functioning), "basic symptoms" (thought interference, disturbance of receptive language, and visual perception disturbance), attenuated or subthreshold psychotic symptoms, neurocognitive deficits, and neurobiological changes measured via magnetic resonance imaging (MRI). Increasing improvements in the identification of those truly at "high risk" for psychotic disorder have paved the way of early intervention strategies in this population and increased the possibility of minimizing distress and disability and delaying or even preventing the onset of an evident psychotic disorder. The treatment (antipsychotic medication, psychological and social interventions) for young people who meet ARMS criteria should not only focus on the symptoms that constitute the ARMS criteria but also address the broader range of difficulties with which the young person might present. There are some ethical issues to consider when selecting specific treatment options, and the potential risks of treatment have to be balanced against the potential benefits.

Keywords: early recognition, clinical staging model, prodromal phase, at risk mental state, prevention

1. Introduction

Schizophrenia is a heterogenous disorder presenting as episodes of psychosis against a background of cognitive, social, and functional impairments.

Schizophrenia, a multifaceted neuropsychiatric disorder, is affecting approximately 1% of the population worldwide. Its onset is the result of a complex interplay of genetic predisposition and environmental factors.

IntechOpen

After more than 100 years of studies and clinical psychiatric practice, passing through numerous conceptualizations of psychosis and schizophrenia, research tries to achieve an evolutionary pattern of psychosis and to establish clear, distinctive diagnostic criteria for every type of psychosis.

Psychosis is unanimously considered essential for understanding the evolution and treatment process and also for estimation of prognosis.

Recently, the area of "prodromal" research in schizophrenia and related disorders has grown considerably. From initial retrospective studies of this phase, dating back to the early twentieth century, the last decade of the century has seen the beginning and expansion of prospective studies aiming to identify the earliest manifestations of psychotic illnesses. From identification of these prodromal or "ultrahigh-risk"(UHR) individuals, the area has also developed to include intervention studies aiming to prevent, delay, or ameliorate the onset of a full-blown psychotic disorder and to investigate underlying processes that cause or contribute to the onset [1].

The fact that psychosis disorders, such as schizophrenia, begin with a prodromal phase prior to the onset of frank psychotic symptoms has been known since the first description of the illness was documented [1].

The pattern of psychosis and of the first episode of psychosis is similar to the pattern of schizophrenia but more complex.

Strauss and Carpenter considered that schizophrenia includes an interactive, developmental, and systematic model [2–6]. By analogy, the model of the first psychotic episode can be considered an interactive, developmental, and systematic model.

The arguments to sustain this theory (hypothesis) are:

1. Variables that interact either sequentially or simultaneously and are nonspecific or partly known.

2. Genetic vulnerability is sometimes well known; in the first psychotic episode, there is a variety of genetic mechanisms with varying degrees of impact and strong expressiveness even from the prodromal or prepsychotic period. But for those with well-known genetic vulnerability, clinical expressivity may be missing, and not everyone with genetic predisposition shows schizophrenia.

3. Perinatal factors may constitute an independent variable that increases the person's vulnerability to develop a psychotic pathology, and when interacting with genetic and environmental factors, the risk increases both in schizophrenia and psychosis [7].

Due to the complexity and heterogeneity of the first psychotic episode, to conceive and to unanimously recognize it like a coherent and unitary model are extremely difficult. The unknowns of this huge puzzle are still numerous despite the scientific efforts.

The model of the first psychotic episode has a medium- or long-term impact on schizophrenia model and can be of particular relevance to both etiopathogenesis and treatment as well as prevention strategies.

Over the last years, the most exciting signs of progress in defining a new conceptualization of psychosis are reported by the genomic studies [8, 9]. Maps of the neurobiological circuits of cognitive functions have been designed and have tried to explain the ways in which these circuits become dysfunctional in various disorders including the psychotic ones.

2. Description of psychosis

Researchers from the National Institute of Mental Health (NIMH) have reported three conclusions:

1. Psychosis is a neurodevelopmental disorder, with onset in adolescence and period when the cortex is still in development.

2. For most disorders related to the cortical functions, the changes of cognitive and comportamental fields appear (occur) later, suggesting the existence of biological dysfunctions long before psychosis.

3. Psychosis like other complex diseases has a multifactorial determinism.

These data have facilitated the explanations of the pattern of psychosis by integrating molecular biology, neuroscience, and behavioral sciences. This new approach tries to discover finally the new treatment strategies including new medications (antipsychotics) and psychological, social, and other potential interventions.

The work group for psychosis within DSM-V proposes distinct clinical domains for each psychotic disorder correlated with the neuronal circuits [10].

In 2009 Jim van Os, one of the members of work group for psychosis, proposed a new syndrome named "salience dysregulation syndrome" as a diagnostic to be used [11].

Jim van Os used the psychotic model of Kapur who considers that hallucinations and delusional ideas appear because the individual has difficulties in recognizing his or her mental experience relevance. Jim van Os used the term syndrome not disease, because a syndrome is a set of symptoms that appear simultaneous without having a common cause. The symptoms described are positive and negative symptoms, disorganization, developmental cognitive deficits, and depressive and maniacal symptoms [11].

The "salience dysregulation syndrome" was divided for diagnosis into:

a. "Salience dysregulation syndrome with developmental cognitive deficits"

b. "Salience dysregulation syndrome with affective expression"

c. "Salience dysregulation syndrome not otherwise specified" [11]

3. Attenuated syndrome

In 2010, Dominguez and collaborators [12] also members of work group for psychosis described two new innovative aspects:

- Deconstructing psychosis/schizophrenia disorganization considered as a syndrome.

- The attenuation of psychotic symptoms is a favorable predictor for the outcome.

In his study [12], Dominguez considered that the association of negative symptoms or of the disorganization with attenuated psychotic symptoms increases the risk of developing a psychotic frank syndrome.

4. The prodrome

Although there is great variability between patients in how their prodromes manifest, certain symptoms and signs have been frequently described. These include depressed mood, anxiety, irritability and aggressive behavior, suicidal ideation and attempts, and substance use. The most commonly occurring prodromal symptoms, according to retrospective studies of patients with schizophrenia and schizophreniform disorder, are reduced concentration and attention, reduced drive and motivation, depression, sleep disturbance, social withdrawal, suspiciousness, deterioration in role functioning, and irritability [1].

Studying these symptoms, we observe two things. First, many of them are nonspecific occurring frequently in the prodromes of nonpsychotic threshold syndromes. Second, a considerable amount of psychiatric symptoms, disability, self-harming, and other health-damaging behaviors, occur during this prodromal phase, even in the earliest stages [1, 19, 22, 39].

Cognitive, affective, and social disturbances known as "basic symptoms" are also commonly described in the early prodromal phases. This concept of "basic symptoms," developed in the 1960s, has significantly influenced the new area of prodromal research [1].

5–10% of the general population experience attenuated or subthreshold form of psychotic symptoms like transient perceptual symptoms; suspiciousness; reference and bizarre delusional ideas (e.g., the beliefs that others may be thinking badly about or laughing at); nonattendance at school, university, or work; and altered behavior toward family and friends [1, 16].

The difference between these phenomena and clear psychotic symptoms is due to their intensity, frequency, duration, and deleterious effects on the individual functionality of the person.

Neurocognitive deficits in particular impaired attention, spatial and verbal memory, and speeded information processing are also evident in the prodromal phase but at a lower degree of severity comparing to those found in first-degree relatives of patients with schizophrenia or in fully affected patients [1].

Specific cognitive deficits may be related more directly to affected brain structures and candidate genes and so may be more directly predictive of psychosis.

5. Treatment

In the prodromal and in the onset phase of psychosis, neurobiological changes can be identified. During the process of transition to psychosis, magnetic resonance imaging (MRI) highlights significant bilateral reduction in gray matter volume in the cingulate region as well as in the left parahippocampal gyrus, left fusiform gyrus, left orbitofrontal cortex, and one region of the left cerebellar cortex [1]. It is important to notify that these brain changes were not present in the UHR group that did not develop psychosis.

The differentiation between normal and abnormal has important implications for defining the prodromal phase of schizophrenia and the therapeutic interventions at this early stage. Atypical antipsychotics has improved the treatment and the outcome of schizophrenia and psychosis due to their low risk for adverse effects like extrapyramidal effects, tardive dyskinesia, sedation, weight gain, metabolic syndrome, amenorrhea, galactorrhea, sexual dysfunctions, etc.

Psychosocial interventions give optimism regarding the prognosis of disease by improving family and social difficulties, stigma avoidance, victimization, isolation, and poverty [13].

If the prodrome can be recognized prospectively and treatment can be provided at this stage, then disability could be minimized, some recovery may be possible before symptoms and poor functioning become obvious, and the possibility of preventing is feasible and realistic. The early intervention aims:

- To slow or possibly to stop further deterioration and even further progression to psychosis.
- To reduce the poor functional outcome characterizing many vulnerable individuals, whether or not psychosis actually develops.
- To evaluate and prevent secondary morbidity in order to decrease morbidity and mortality in the first episode of psychosis.
- To create research opportunities to develop new therapeutic strategies.
- To develop secondary prevention strategies.

Early intervention has to take place in the three important phases of early psychosis:

a. In the phase of risk when the symptoms are subtle and can be confused with particularities and difficulties specific to adolescence.

b. In the period of frank psychosis in which if the symptoms remain untreated, there is a risk of temporal or permanent disability.

c. In the critical period after the onset of the first episode of psychosis, a period which can last up to 5 years after the onset, the length of time that treatment should be comprehensive and specific.

6. Redefining psychosis

The latest attempts redefining the concept of psychosis have focused particularly on the first episode of psychosis and on prodromal stage of schizophrenia.

Arguments for these new concepts can be synthesized as:

- Clinical heterogeneity of patients diagnosed with first psychotic episode.
- The heterogenous outcome of these patients.
- The instability of the diagnosis over time.
- Avoidance of negative prognostic.
- Stigma avoidance.

7. A history of prodrome: benefits of diagnosis of the prodrome

Over 100 years ago, Emil Kraepelin (1896), cited by Patrick McGorry at the beginning of the chapter "A stitch in time" [14], wrote "it is of the greatest medical importance to diagnose cases of dementia praecox certainly and at an early stage" (Kraepelin, 1896/1987, p. 23).

In 1908, Eugen Bleuler, cited by Patrick McGorry in the same book [14], wrote "the sooner the patients can be recovered and the less they are allowed to withdraw in their own world, the sooner they become socially functional" (Bleuler, 1908/1987, p. 63).

Coming from 1927 [15], we find the same idea "I feel certain that many incipient cases might be arrested before the efficient contact with reality is completely suspended, and a long stay in institutions made necessary" ([15], p. 135). Meares in 1950 wrote "it is not necessary to diagnose early schizophrenia but to diagnose prepsychotic schizophrenia ,to prevent damage".

These statements can be used not only as the foundation stones for any therapeutic intervention but also as arguments to emphasize the importance of early phases of psychosis.

8. Definition of prodrome

So, the prodrome is a distinct period in the evolution of the first psychotic episode, mostly unknown or minimized as importance. The onset's particularities and the evolution of the first psychotic episode are involved in the short-, medium-, and long-term prognosis. The recovery depends on the early initiation of therapeutic strategies.

The prodrome was originally defined as the prepsychotic period preceding a relapse in patients already diagnosed with psychosis. Subsequently a distinction was made between the initial and the relapse prodrome [16].

Other definitions are [16]:

- "a heterogenous group of behaviors having a temporal relationship with psychosis' onset".
- "the period from the first symptoms noted until the onset of prominent psychotic symptoms".

All definitions of prodrome phase have in common the presence of symptoms and the temporal relationship with the onset of psychosis, with two important practical consequences. The first implication is the person being symptomatic during the prodrome will ask for medical help, so it is possible to establish a diagnosis and a therapeutic strategy. The second implication is the person can develop the disease after the end of the prodromal phase, suggesting that the transition from prodrome to frank psychosis may be detectable.

9. False positives and treatment

However, early attempts at prodromal intervention were hampered, by the problem of "false positives" and their implications for preventive intervention. "False positives" refer to those who are identified as being prodromal, at risk of developing a psychotic disorder in the near future, but who do not do so. Some of these people were in fact never "destined" to develop a psychotic disorder (the "true false positives") [1]. These persons may be harmed by being considered as "prodromal" or "high risk of psychosis" and may receive treatment unnecessarily

[17–19]. In contrast are those individuals who would have developed a psychotic disorder were it not for some alteration in their circumstances,such as a treatment intervention, stress reduction or cessation of illicit drug use, that preventing this form occurring [1]. This latter group has been termed "false false positive" [19]. It is virtually impossible to distinguish between these two groups phenotypically at baseline and follow-up.

10. Description of prodromal phase

The conceptualization of the prodrome phase uses two methods: a retrospective/passive method which involves getting information from the patient and his/her family and a proactive one which includes observation and patient monitoring during psychosis.

Yung and McGorry [16] describe the phenomenology of the prodrome phase, summarizing the data from the literature with those of the Melbourne Personal Assessment and Crisis Evaluation (PACE) approach [20, 21]. The PACE Clinic recruits those patients with a perceived need for psychiatric help.

11. Ultrahigh risk

The PACE ultrahigh-risk (UHR) criteria require that a young person aged between 14 and 30 is referred for health care to the clinic if the criteria for one or more of the following groups are met:

1. Attenuated psychotic symptom (APS) group has experienced subthreshold, attenuated positive psychotic symptoms during the past year.

2. Brief limited intermittent psychotic symptom (BLIPS) group has experienced episodes of frank psychotic symptoms that have not lasted longer than a week and have spontaneously abated.

3. Trait and state risk factor group has a first-degree relative with a psychotic disorder or the identified subject with a schizotypal personality disorder and has experienced a significant decrease in functioning during the previous year [19, 22]

The ultrahigh-risk (UHR) criteria allow the recognition of young people at risk of onset of a psychotic disorder (late adolescence/early adulthood) who also report mental state disorder suggesting an emerging psychotic process or who may have a positive family history of psychosis accompanied by evidence of mental ill health.

Necessarily, criteria have also been developed to define the onset of frank psychosis. These are not identical to DSM-V criteria [22, 23] but are elaborated to define the minimal point at which antipsychotic treatment is indicated. This definition is arbitrary but even has a well-defined treatment implication, applicable equally to "substance-related symptoms, symptoms that have a mood component—either depression or mania—and schizophrenia spectrum disorders." The predictive aim is the first-episode psychosis requiring antipsychotic treatment, arbitrarily defined by the persistence of clear psychotic symptoms, more than 1 week [1, 19].

The intensity of psychotic symptoms characteristic for each of the UHR groups was firstly assessed using the following scales: the "Brief Psychiatric Rating Scale (BPRS) and the Comprehensive Assessment of Symptoms and History (CASH) interview." To specify the frequency and duration of psychotic symptoms, new criteria were needed. So, a new instrument, the Comprehensive Assessment of At Risk Mental States (CAARMS) was designed so that all relevant domains (intensity, frequency, duration, and recency) could be assessed [1, 24].

The PACE UHR criteria have been adopted and adapted in a large number of other settings around the world (USA, UK, Norway, Germany, etc.).

Symptoms associated with prodromal phase.

Yung and McGorry [16] identified eight subtypes of symptoms characteristic of prodromal phase:

- Neurotic symptoms: anxiety, irritability, restlessness.

- Affective symptoms: depression, anhedonia, guilt, suicidal ideas, thymic oscillations.

- Volitional disturbances: apathy, loss of interest, low energy, fatigue.

- Cognitive deficits: attention deficit, rumination, abstraction difficulties, thought blockages, thought interference, thought perseveration, thought pressure.

- Psychotic symptoms: visual and auditory perceptual disturbances, suspiciousness or paranoid ideation, derealization, unstable ideas of reference.

- Physical symptoms: somatic symptoms, weight loss, low appetite, sleeping disorders.

- Behavioral dysfunctions: social withdrawal, impulsivity, aggressivity, bizarre behavior, functional deterioration.

- Other symptoms: sensitivity, odd beliefs or magical thinking, dissociation.

Yung and collaborators [19, 25] have elaborated a set of operational criteria to identify individuals at risk for developing a psychotic disorder over the next 6–24 months as Global Assessment of Functioning (GAF) scale score <51, BPRS score >2, and Hamilton Depression Rating Scale (HRDS) score >18 [19, 25].

12. Risk factors to developing psychosis

During the years, several research teams have identified a number of risk factors for the development of psychosis: Carr and collaborators (2000): family history, perinatal complications, premorbid personality, stressful life events; Mason et al. [26]: schizotypal personality disorder, hallucinations, magic thinking, odd beliefs, anhedonia, withdrawal, functional deterioration [27].

13. Duration of prodrome

Regarding the duration of the prodrome, retrospective studies suggest a variation ranging from a short period to several years [7, 26, 28].

14. Genetic risk programs for psychosis

The development of genetic high-risk (GHR) programs was an important step for early detection and intervention, especially in schizophrenia.

In recent years, genetic research have identified specific genes for schizophrenia, some with early phenotypic expression may be considered important biomarkers, for example, the CHRNA7 gene situated on chromosome 15 with importance in genetic transmission and heredity of schizophrenia [29–32].

The phenotype "schizophrenia" has been characterized by the presence of behavioral abnormalities, the related outcome, and its longitudinal course, but not its fundamental biological substrate. The absence of a neuropathological basis for schizophrenia was one reason that some researchers supported the neurodevelopmental hypothesis of schizophrenia issued by Weinberger [33]. Evidence of obstetrical complications being associated with the risk of schizophrenia supported that developmental abnormalities were involved [34].

The premorbid risk factors associated with schizophrenia as motor and cognitive delay and obstetrical complications are nonspecific; their prevalence in the non-affected population is important, so their positive predictive value for the development of schizophrenia is limited.

Neuroimaging anomalies found in patients diagnosed with first-episode psychosis have been interpreted as supportive of a static structural abnormality associated with schizophrenia that had originated early in neurodevelopment [35].

Recently, the association of molecular genetics with intermediate phenotypes such as cognitive impairment or abnormal brain functioning, as measured with functional neuroimaging, has generated diverse understanding of major psychosis. The combination of different levels may be of particular importance for longitudinal "at risk" studies. These studies can identify individuals who are at true risk of developing major psychosis prior to its full clinical expression, enabling us to treat "at risk" individuals prior to full manifestation of psychosis and prevent its appearance during critical developmental periods such as late adolescence [1, 36].

The measurement of genetic profiles using groups of candidate genes in combination with psychosocial risk factors such as stress and illicit drug use in samples of patients with clinically significant but subthreshold features of psychosis and mood disorder is a key strategy in enhancing predictive power for transition to more established and severe psychotic disorders, in treatment selection, and in longer-term prognosis [1].

Genetic studies suggest that diagnostic boundaries may be modified based on genetic information and some genes such as NRG1, DTNBP1, DISC1, and BDNF may relate to risk for both schizophrenia and mood disorders [37]. The synergistic use of genotyping with phenotypes characterizing brain functioning will contribute to a better understanding of the mechanisms by which genes interact with other genes and/or environmental risk factors.

15. Disadvantages of "prodromal" identification

Identification by different methods of people at risk of psychosis in the general population has allowed an increase in accuracy from a rate of 1% to a rate of approximately 30% [1]. However, the increase in accuracy has raised some criticism. One is that the screening would not be effective in the general population because of the lower base rate of psychotic illness in that population [38], so screening for UHR criteria would not be supported at this stage [19]. The second criticism is that there is a high false positive rate in all of these studies, the majority of participants not developing psychotic disorder. Consequently, some persons will be "diagnosed" and treated as if they were at "high risk" of psychosis, when this may not be true. This false identification may have negative consequences on those individuals: they may become anxious or depressed about the possibility of developing schizophrenia or receiving treatment, stigmatized by others or themselves or both [39]. These people may be exposed to drug or other therapies, with potential adverse effects without gaining any benefit [39, 40–43]. This controversy on the risk benefit balance of early intervention strategies must be addressed by future studies.

16. Predictors of psychotic disorder in high-risk groups

Since 2004, many prospective programs focused on early psychoses have been developed.

The term "at risk mental state" (ARMS) is still used today to describe individuals at risk to develop a psychotic disorder [1, 44]. So, different diagnostic systems have been achieved, one of the most known and sophisticated systems being developed by McGorry and his team (1966) in order to reduce the number of "false positive" cases [1, 44]. The diagnostic system accomplished by McGorry et al. has three categories of diagnostic criteria for individuals' "at risk mental state" (ARMS):

1. Attenuated psychotic symptoms (APS).

    a. The presence of at least one of the following: ideas of reference, odd beliefs, magical thinking, perception disturbances, paranoid ideation, formal thought disorder, disturbances of receptive language.

    b. Frequency of symptoms: several times a week.

    c. Duration: have experienced subthreshold, attenuated positive psychotic symptoms during the past year.

    d. Recently: stressful life events during the last year.

2. Brief limited intermittent psychotic symptoms group (BLIPS).

    a. Transient psychotic symptoms: the presence of at least one of the following—ideas of reference, odd beliefs, magical thinking, perception disturbances, paranoid ideation, formal thought disorder, disturbances of receptive language.

    b. Frequency of symptoms: few times a week.

    c. Duration: less than a week and spontaneously abated.

    d. Recently: short intermittent psychotic symptoms were present during the previous year.

3. Trait and state risk factor group.

    a. First-degree relative with a psychotic disorder or the identified individual with a schizotypal personality disorder.

b. Significant decline in functioning during the previous year.

c. Duration: at least 1 month and no more than 5 years [19, 22].

These criteria were criticized for the absence of negative symptoms of schizophrenia.

Cornblatt et al. mentioned, among the diagnostic criteria of the prodrome, negative attenuated symptoms or disorganization, which define clinical high-risk (CHR) group representing the early prodromal stage and CHRT group representing tardive prodromal stage [45]. CHRT group is characterized by negative attenuated symptoms, disorganization, and positive symptoms.

Negative symptoms are impaired concentration and attention, subjectively abnormal emotional experiences, blunted affect, impaired energy, and impaired tolerance to stress [24].

Marked impairment in role functioning, flat or inappropriate affect, anhedonia, and asociality were found at significantly higher levels at baseline in those who went on to develop psychosis than in those who did not [26]. So, negative symptoms have been found to be predictive of psychosis [1].

Positive symptoms like unusual thought content, suspiciousness, perceptual disturbance, conceptual disorganization, and disorganized communication are significant predictors of psychosis [19, 46, 47].

The ultrahigh-risk (UHR) criteria have been used and modified in different countries around the world: USA, UK, Germany, and Finland.

The German Research Network on Schizophrenia (GNRS), Cologne, Bonn, Düsseldorf, and Munich, introduced the basic symptoms into the definition on the prodrome [48, 49].

The basic symptoms included thought interferences, perseveration, pressure or blockages, and disturbances of receptive language; decreased ability to discriminate between ideas and perception or fantasy and true memories; unstable ideas of reference; derealization; and visual or auditory perceptual disturbances. Using these basic symptoms, it should be possible to identify subjects at risk of developing schizophrenia, and so early intervention is possible. Because basic symptoms were frequently found before any subthreshold or attenuated psychotic symptoms, these criteria were thought to be detecting the very beginning of the initial prodromal phase [50].

Unlike McGorry et al., the GNRS distinguishes between the "early initial prodromal state" (EIPS) and the "late initial prodromal state" (LIPS). The EIPS criteria attempt to define a group at incipient but not imminent or immediate risk of psychosis. The criteria consist of the 10 predictive basic symptoms of which one or more is required, plus the PACE trait and state risk UHR criterion.

16.1 The EIPS criteria

One or more of the following basic symptoms:

- Thinking disturbances: perseveration, pressure, blockage, ideas of reference (unstable)
- Disturbances of visual and auditory perception
- Disturbances of receptive language (either heard or read)
- Diminished capacity to discern between ideas and perception, fantasy, and true memory

16.2 Derealization

The onset of the symptoms has occurred at least a year ago, with a frequency of several times a week within the last 3 months.

- Decrease in "the Global Assessment Functioning Score" (DSM-V) of at least 30 points in the past year which add one of the following risk factors: "first-degree relative with a lifetime diagnosis of schizophrenia or a schizophrenia spectrum disorder and/or pre- or perinatal complications".

- The absence of attenuated or transient psychotic symptoms [1].

The LIPS criterion attempts to identify those at more immediate risk and is based on the APS and BLIPS criteria [51].

16.3 The LIPS criteria

- The presence of at least one of the following attenuated positive symptoms (APS) present within the last 3 months, appearing several times per week for a period of at least 1 week, but no longer in the same severity than 1 year: "ideas of reference; odd beliefs or magical thinking; unusual perceptual experiences; odd thinking or speech; suspiciousness or paranoid ideation".

- "Brief limited intermittent psychotic symptoms (BLIPS), defined as appearance of one of the following frank psychotic symptoms for less than 1 week (interval between episodes at least 1 week) and resolving spontaneously: hallucinations; delusions; formal thought disorder; gross disorganized or catatonic behaviour" [1].

This two-stage prodromal state guides the treatment approach, that is, psychological or pharmacological therapy [51–53]. LIPS criteria denote an imminent risk of transition to psychotic disorder within the next 12 months, so an antipsychotic medication—second generation—appeared justified. Psychological interventions were crisis intervention, psychoeducation, family counseling, and assistance with education or work-related difficulties.

In EIPS group the psychological intervention (cognitive behavioral therapy (CBT) or the supportive control condition) appeared successful in preventing further progression of the illness [54].

17. Early intervention and prevention

Early intervention may be able to delay or even prevent onset of psychosis in the UHR or prodromal stage. Both antipsychotic medication (risperidone 1–2 mg/day, olanzapine 5–15 mg/day) and psychological interventions (cognitive behavioral therapy (CBT), case management, supportive therapy, problem-solving strategies) might have a role in treating the difficulties and problems that UHR young people experience, as well as in reducing the rate of transition to psychosis and in reducing symptomatology. Deterioration in psychosocial functioning and persistent disability is also an important treatment goal [1].

Therapeutic strategies must be personalized and correlated with the first psychotic episode stages. Treatment for young people who meet ARMS criteria should not only focus on the symptoms that constitute the ARMS criteria but also address the range of difficulties which the young person might present.

Side effects associated with all antipsychotic medications are weight gain, diabetes, and sexual dysfunction for olanzapine [55–57] and sexual dysfunction and insomnia for risperidone [1]. Extrapyramidal side effects such as tardive dyskinesia, which is often irreversible, are less common with the newer, atypical antipsychotics [58, 59]. Evidence also suggests that certain antipsychotics (haloperidol) reduced gray matter volume in the brains of patients with a first episode of psychosis [60]. In contrast the newer second-generation antipsychotic medications, in fact, have neuroprotective qualities.

Antipsychotic drugs are potentially useful in the latter phases of the prodromal period when attenuated psychotic symptoms are evident and the individual is on the edge of a conversion to full psychosis.

Psychological interventions are useful in earlier and less symptomatic stages of the prodrome, to manage the stress, depression, anxiety, sleep disturbance, and decline in functioning. CBT should be effective for people with attenuated psychotic symptoms or with brief limited intermittent psychotic symptoms and for individuals who are "false positives" [22].

Psychological treatments may be not only necessary but sufficient for some of these putatively prodromal patients [1].

Further researches are required to determine which treatment strategies are most effective and how long they should be continued.

Ethical considerations associated with treatment of young people who meet ARMS criteria have been widely debated [17, 28, 40, 41, 42, 45, 46]. Concerns about stigma associated with being identified as having a label of ARMS "false positives" and for how long should treatment be provided (in other words, how long is the period of risk) remain unresolved, and even clinical research into ARMS has now been conducted for over a decade.

Author details

Delia Marina Podea[1*], Romina Teodora Moldovan[2] and Laura Cristina Popa[3]

1 Personal Medical Center for Psychiatry "Dr. Podea Delia", Arad, Romania

2 Emergency Clinical County Hospital of Arad, "Victor Babes" University of Medicine and Pharmacy, Timisoara, Romania

3 Emergency Clinical County Hospital of Arad, "Carol Davila" University of Medicine and Pharmacy, Bucharest, Romania

*Address all correspondence to: deliapodea@yahoo.com

References

[1] Jackson HJ, McGorry PD. The Recognition and Management of Early Psychosis. A Preventive Approach. 2nd ed. Cambridge University Press; 2009

[2] Kirkpatrick B, Buchanan RW, Ross DE, Carpenter WT. A separate disease within the syndrome of schizophrenia. Archives of General Psychiatry. 2001;**58**:165-171

[3] BuchananRW,CarpenterWT.Domains of psychopathology: An approach to the reduction of heterogeneity in schizophrenia. Journal of Nervous and Mental Disorders. 1994;**182**:193-204

[4] Strauss JS, Carpenter WT. Schizophrenia. New York: Plenum Publishing Corporation; 1981

[5] Strauss JS, Carpenter WT Jr, Bartko JJ. The diagnosis and understanding schizophrenic symptoms and signs. Schizophrenia Bulletin. 1974;**11**:61-69

[6] Strauss JS. Subjectivity and severe psychiatric disorders. Schizophrenia Bulletin. 2001;**37**(1):8-13

[7] Sharma T, Harvey PD. The Early Course of Schizophrenia. Oxford University Press; 2006

[8] Owen MJ, Craddock N, Jablensky A. The genetic deconstruction of psychosis. Schizophrenia Bulletin. 2007;**33**:905-911

[9] Taminga CA, Sirovatkan PJ, Regier DA, van Os J. Deconstructing Psychosis. Refining the Research Agenda for DSM V. American Psychiatric Association; 2010

[10] Cuthbert BN, Insel TR. Toward new approaches to psychotic disorders: The NIMH Research Domain Criteria Project. Schizophrenia Bulletin. 2010;**36**(6):1061-1062

[11] Van Os J. A silence dysregulation syndrome. The British Journal of Psychiatry. 2009;**194**:101-103

[12] Dominguez MDG, Saka MC, Lieb R, Wittchen HU, Van Os J. Early expression of negative/disorganized symptoms predicting psychotic experiences and subsequent clinical psychosis: A 10-year study. The American Journal of Psychiatry. 2010;**167**:1075-1082

[13] Tacchi MJ, Scott J. Improving Adherence in Schizophrenia and Bipolar Disorders. The Atrium, Southern Gate, Chichester, West Sussex: John Wiley and Sons; 2005

[14] McGorry PD, Jackson HJ. The Recognition and Management of Early Psychosis: A Preventive Approach. Cambridge University Press; 2004

[15] Sullivan HS. The onset of schizophrenia. American Journal of Psychiatry. 1994;**151**:135-139

[16] Yung AR, McGorry PD. The prodromal phase of the first episode psychosis: Past and current conceptualisations. Schizophrenia Bulletin. 1996;**22**:353-370

[17] Corcoran C, Malaspina D, Hercher L. Prodromal interventions for schizophrenia vulnerability: The risks of being "AT RISK". Schizophrenia Research. 2005;**73**:173-184

[18] Heinssen S, Bowen J, Emmani J, et al. A one year prospective study of the effects of life events and medication in the etiology of schizophrenic relapse. British Journal of Psychiatry. 1996;**168**:49-56

[19] Yung AR, Phillips LJ, Yuen HP, et al. Psychosis prediction: 12 month follow up of a high-risk ("prodromal") group. Schizophrenia Research. 2003;**6**:21-32

[20] Yung AR, McGorry PD, McFarlane CA, Patton G. The pace clinic- development of clinical service for young people at high risk of psychosis. Australian Psychiatry. 1995;**3**:345-349

[21] Young AR, McGorry PD. Monitoring and care of young people at incipient risk of psychosis. Schizophrenia Bulletin. 1996;**22**:283-303

[22] Yung AR, Phillips LJ, McGorry PD. Treating Schizophrenia in the Prodromal Phase. London: Dunitz; 2004

[23] APA. Diagnostic and Statistical Manual of Mental Disorders. 5th ed. American Psychiatric Publishing; 2013

[24] Young AR, Yuen HP, McGorry PD, et al. Mapping the onset of psychosis: The comprehensive assessment of at risk mental states (CAARMS). Australian and New Zeeland Journal of Psychiatry. 2005;**39**:964-971

[25] Yung AR, Phillips LJ, McGorry PD, et al. Prediction of psychosis. A step towards indicated prevention of schizophrenia. The British Journal of Psychiatry. Supplement. 1998;**172**(33):14-20

[26] Mason O et al. Risk factors for transition to first episode psychosis, among individuals with at-risk mental states. Schizophrenia Research. 2004;**71**:227-237

[27] Perkins D. Evaluating and treating the prodromal stage of schizophrenia. Current Psychiatry Reports. 2004;**6**:289

[28] Phillips LJ, McGorry PD, Yung AR, McGlashan TH, et al. Prepsychotic phase of schizophrenia and related disorders: Recent progress and future opportunities. British Journal of Psychiatry. 2005;**187**:33-44

[29] Philips LJ, Yung R, McGorry PD. Identification of young people at risk of psychosis: Validation of personal assessment and crisis evaluation clinic intake criteria. Australian and New Zealand Journal of Psychiatry. 2000;**34**:164-169

[30] Kendler KS, Diehl SR. The genetics of schizophrenia: A current, genetic-epidemiologic perspective. Schizophrenia Bulletin. 1993;**19**:261-285

[31] Stefanis NC, Van OSJ, Avramopoulos D, et al. Variation in catechol-o-methyltransferase val158 met genotype associated with schizotypy but not recognition: A population study in 543 young men. Biological Psychiatry. 2004;**56**:510-515

[32] Freedman R et al. Early biomarkers of psychosis. Dialogues in Clinical Neuroscience. 2005;**7**:17-12

[33] Weinberger DR. Implications of normal brain development for the pathogenesis of schizophrenia. Archives of General Psychiatry. 1987;**44**:660-669

[34] Murray RM, Lewis SW. Is schizophrenia a neurodevelopmental disorder? British Medical Journal (Clinical Research Edition). 1987;**295**:681-682

[35] Weinberger DR, McClure RK. Neurotoxicity, neuroplasticity and magnetic resonance imaging morphometry. What is happening in the schizophrenic brain? Archives of General Psychiatry. 2002;**59**:553-558

[36] Yung AR, Yuen HP, Berger G, et al. Declining transition rate in ultra high risk (prodromal) services: Dilution or reduction of risk? Schizophrenia Bulletin. 2002;**33**:673-681

[37] Prathikanti S, Weinberger DR. Psychiatric genetics—The New Era: Genetic research and some clinical implications. British Medical Bulletin. 2005;**73-74**:107-122

[38] Warner R. Problems with early and very early intervention in psychosis. British Journal of Psychiatry. 2005;**48**:104-107

[39] Yung AR, Phillips LJ, Yuen HP, McGorry PD. Risk factors for psychosis in an ultra high risk group. Psychopathology and clinical features. Schizophrenia Research. 2004;**67**:131-142

[40] Cornblatt BA, Lencz T, Kane JM. Treatment of the schizophrenia prodrome: It is presently ethical? Schizophrenia Research. 2001;**51**:31-38

[41] McGlashan TH. Psychosis treatment prior to psychosis onset: Ethical issues. Schizophrenia Research. 2001;**51**:47-54

[42] McGorry PD, Yung A, Phillips L. Ethics and early interventions in psychosis: Keeping up the PACE and staying in step. Schizophrenia Research. 2001;**51**:17-29

[43] Yung AR, McGorry PD. Is the pre-psychotic intervention realistic in schizophrenia and related disorders? Australian and New Zealand Journal of Psychiatry. 1997;**31**:799-805

[44] McGorry PD. The recognition and optimal management of early detection and optimal management of early psychosis: An evidence based reform. World Psychiatry. 2002:76-83

[45] Cornblatt BA, Lencz T, Smith CW, et al. The schizophrenia prodrome revised: A neurodevelopmental perspective. Schizophrenia Bulletin. 2003;**29**:633-651

[46] Haroun N, Dunn L, Haroun A, Cadenhead K. Risk and protection in prodromal schizophrenia: Ethical implication for clinical practice and future research. Schizophrenia Bulletin. 2006;**32**:166-178

[47] Miller TJ, McGlashan TH, Rosen JL, et al. Prospective diagnosis of the initial prodrome for schizophrenia based on the structured interview for prodromal syndromes: Preliminary evidence of interrater reliability and predictive variability. American Journal of Psychiatry. 2002;**159**:863-865

[48] Hafner H, Maurer K, Ruhrmann S, et al. Early detection and secondary prevention of psychosis: Facts and visions. European Archives of Psychiatry and Clinical Neuroscience. 2004;**254**:117-128

[49] Wolver W, Buchkremer G, Hafner H, et al. German research/ network on schizophrenia. Bridging the gap between research and care. European Archive of Psychiatry and Clinical Neuroscience. 2003;**253**:321-329

[50] Hafner H, Maurer W, Loffler B, et al. Onset and early course of schizophrenia. In: Hafner H, Gattaz WF, editors. Search of the Causes of Schizophrenia. New York: Springer; 1995. pp. 43-66

[51] Ruhrmann S, Schultze-Lutter F, Klosterkotter J. Early detection and intervention in the initial prodromal phase of schizophrenia. Pharmacopsychiatry. 2003;**36**(Suppl):162-167

[52] Bechdolf A, Ruhrmann S, Wagner M, et al. Interventions in the initial prodromal states of psychosis in Germany: Concept and recruitment. British Journal of Psychiatry. 2005;**187**:45-48. (Special issues: Early psychosis a bridge to the future)

[53] Ruhrmann S, Schultze-Lutter F, Maier W, Klosterkotter J. Pharmacological intervention in the initial prodromal phase of psychosis. European Psychiatry. 2005;**20**:1-6

[54] Bechdolf A, Philips LJ, Francey SM, et al. Recent approaches to psychological

intervention for people at risk of psychosis. European Archives of Psychiatry and Clinical Neuroscience. 2006;**256**:159-173

[55] Eder-Ischia U, Ebenbiuchler C, Fleischhacker WW. Olanzapine induced weight gain and disturbances of lipid and glucose metabolism. Essential Psychopharmacology. 2005;**6**:112-117

[56] Kinon BJ, Kaiser CJ, Ahmed S, Rotelli MD, Kollack-Walker S. Association between early and rapid weight gain and change in weight over one year of olanzapine therapy in patients with schizophrenia and related disorders. Journal of Clinical Psychopharmacology. 2005;**25**:255-258

[57] Newcomer JW. Second generation (atypical) antipsychotics and metabolic effects: A comprehensive literature review. CNS Drugs. 2005;**19**(suppl 1):1-93

[58] Kane JM. Tardive dyskinesia rates with atypical antipsychotics in adults: Prevalence and incidence. Journal of Clinical Psychiatry. 2004;**65**(suppl 9): 16-20

[59] Margolese HC, Chouinard G, Kolivakis TT, et al. Tardive dyskinesia in the area of typical and atypical antipsychotics. Part 2: Incidence and management strategies in patients with schizophrenia. Canadian Journal of Psychiatry. 2005;**50**:703-714

[60] Liberman JA, Tollefson GD, Schulz C, HGDH Study Group. Antipsychotic drug effects on brain morphology in first-episode psychosis. Archives of General Psychiatry. 2005;**62**:361-370

Section 3

Epilepsy, Cerebral Palsy and Ataxia

Chapter 4

Epilepsy and Cerebral Palsy

Boulenouar Mesraoua, Musab Ali, Dirk Deleu, Hassan Al Hail, Gayane Melikyan, Naim Haddad, Osama Alalamy, Covanis Athanasios and Ali A. Asadi-Pooya

Abstract

Abnormalities of muscle tone, movement, and motor skills are the hallmark of cerebral palsy (CP) which results from injury to the developing brain. Clinically, the syndrome evolves over time and may only be apparent after 3–5 years of age, although suggestive signs and symptoms may be present at an earlier age. Epilepsy is common in CP and occurs in about 30% of patients. Generally, the onset is within the first 2 years of life. Epilepsy is commonly observed in children with spastic hemiplegia, followed by quadriplegia and diplegia. Significant risk factors for the development of epilepsy in patients with CP are family history, neonatal seizure, structural abnormalities, low Apgar scores, and mental retardation. Focal to bilateral tonic-clonic seizures are the most prominent seizure types, followed by focal aware or impaired awareness seizures, while infantile spasms and myoclonic jerks are seen in 25% of cases. Mental retardation is a predisposing factor for early onset of seizures and more severe epilepsy. The overall outcome of seizures in children with CP is generally poor, requiring prolonged course of antiepileptic medication, usually polytherapy with higher incidence of refractory seizures, side effects, comorbidities, and hospital admissions for drug-resistant seizures or status epilepticus.

Keywords: cerebral palsy, epilepsy, seizures, treatment, mental retardation

1. Introduction

Cerebral palsy is a term that implies a disorder of motor function. It is a neurodevelopmental abnormality affecting muscle tone, movement, and motor skills. CP is the result of a nonprogressive damage of the nervous system at its early developmental stage and can be caused by several factors encountered in prenatal, perinatal, or postnatal periods [1]. Although the disorder itself is nonprogressive, the clinical expression changes over time as the brain develops and matures.

The International Consensus in 2005 defined CP as follows [2]: "CP is a group of permanent neurological disorders resulting from nonprogressive brain injury or malformation that occurred in the developing fetal or infant brain and primarily affecting body movement, posture and muscle coordination. The motor dysfunction in CP is often associated with abnormal cognitive abilities including communication and behavior, disturbance in sensation and perception and last but not least, epilepsy and secondary musculoskeletal complications".

There is no consensus in the literature about the prevalence of epilepsy in patients with CP. Studies indicate a very wide range of epilepsy in children with CP. However, it is argued that in certain types of CP, higher rate of epilepsy is found and that an average of 30% of patients with CP exhibit seizures. This figure is proportional to the degree of motor and cognitive disabilities [3, 4].

2. Prevalence and incidence of cerebral palsy

The estimated prevalence of CP is approximately 2 per 1000 children. The risk is even higher in preterm infants with low birth weight [5, 6].

The advances in prenatal, perinatal, and postnatal pediatric care significantly influenced the reported incidence and prevalence of CP. The most common causes of CP have varied over time and between geographical locations. While the developed world faces predominantly prematurity and extremely low-birth-weight-related morbidities, the developing countries are still faced with prenatal rubella, perinatal asphyxia, and postnatal hyperbilirubinemia.

From the 1960s to 1980s, the rate of CP and the extent of disability among preterm infants increased as survival improved for the most immature [7]. This trend reversed later, most likely because of improvements in perinatal care [8].

3. Etiology of cerebral palsy

The etiology of CP is multifactorial. Most cases are likely related to prenatal factors: among them prematurity and/or low birth weight. Other associated etiologies include congenital abnormalities, multiple pregnancy, placental pathology, intrauterine infection, metabolic encephalopathies, and genetic forms of CP.

Perinatal hypoxia and ischemia account for only a marginal number of cases of CP. Stroke in the perinatal period may cause CP and is typically manifested as spastic hemiparesis.

In an Australian study of 213 children diagnosed with CP [9], a multifactorial etiology was demonstrated. Major CP-associated pathologies, other than acute intrapartum hypoxia, were found in 98% of cases; some children had several associated pathologies such as

- Prematurity (78%).
- Intrauterine growth restriction (34%).
- Intrauterine infection (28%).
- Antepartum hemorrhage (27%).
- Severe placental pathology (21%).
- Multiple pregnancy (20%).
- Very-low-birth-weight (VLBW) infants (5–15%). In these cases, CP is frequently associated with periventricular leukomalacia, intraventricular hemorrhage, and/or bronchopulmonary dysplasia.

4. Clinical features and classification of cerebral palsy

The classification of CP is based on the type and distribution of motor abnormalities. Suggestive signs and symptoms may be present in infancy, and severe cerebral palsy can be diagnosed as early as 1 month of age. However, the specific CP syndromes are best recognized in time as the child's brain matures, e.g., spastic CP is usually diagnosed after the age of 6 months, dyskinetic CP usually after 18–20 months old, and the ataxic type even later. Following-up the children with high risk will allow early recognition and intervention.

Early diagnosis, in some cases, will enable early intervention for the child by a multidisciplinary team and in addition early psychological and possible financial support to the family.

Early signs of CP include as follows:

Neurobehavioral findings: a neonate who presents with poor feeding with or without recurrent vomiting, irritability, poor sleeping pattern, and poor visual attention should raise suspicion of CP. In addition, prolonged retention or exaggeration of these primitive reflexes is often a premature sign of motor disability. In infants with hyperactive tonic labyrinthine reflex, opisthotonus may occur, or they may roll over at an earlier age than usually expected. Similarly, children with CP may present inadequate posture in vertical suspension in that they present persistent extension of lower extremities on attempting a sitting position.

Motor tone and posture: Tone can be normal in some subjects, but it may be increased or decreased in the extremities of others.

Delay in sitting without support beyond 9 months, poor head control, persistent or asymmetric hand fisting beyond 4 months, and abnormal oromotor patterns (tongue thrusting or grimacing) are often the early motor signs. Sometimes increased neck extensor and axial tone may make head control appears better than it is.

The abovementioned features may also coincide with intellectual impairment, hemianopia, and other visual problems. Also, behavioral problems are frequently found among children with hemiplegic CP including anxiety and specific phobias.

After age 18–24 months, signs and symptoms generally align to a specific subtype of CP:

Spastic CP includes spastic diplegia, spastic hemiplegia, and spastic quadriplegia, with accompanying features pointing to an upper motor neuron syndrome like spastic hypertonia, hyperreflexia, extensor plantar responses, and Dyskinetic CP is characterized by involuntary, stereotyped, uncontrolled, recurring movements of athetosis, chorea, and dystonia.

CP associated with ataxic movements (loss of orderly muscular coordination, unstable gait) and speech is referred to as ataxic CP and is usually associated with a widespread disorder of motor function. Ataxic CP is rare, and children who present with these findings must be evaluated for other potential causes of ataxia.

Mixed CP is a spastic type with ataxic and/or dyskinetic features of variable predominance.

Hypotonic CP is not included in the contemporary classifications. Majority of patients with "hypotonic CP" in early infancy later develop spastic, dyskinetic, or ataxic CP. **Table 1** shows the proportion of the different types of CP.

Spastic subtypes	Percentages (%)
Spastic diplegia	13–25
Spastic hemiplegia	21–40
Spastic quadriplegia	20–43
Dyskinetic subtypes	12–14
Ataxic CP	4–13

Table 1.
Proportion of the different types of cerebral palsy.

5. Associated comorbidities

Besides motor disabilities, there are significant comorbid disorders of cerebral function that may appear or become severe as the child grows including intellectual disability, seizures, behavioral and emotional disorders, speech and language disorders, as well as visual and hearing impairments. Social difficulties and autism spectrum disorders are also commonly associated comorbidities [10]. In addition, many accompanying conditions such as growth failure, pulmonary disease, orthopedic problems (e.g., joint subluxations and dislocations and hip dysplasia), osteopenia, urinary disorders, sleep disturbance, and hypersalivation have been identified. Pain is common in children with CP and can significantly impact the quality of life. Children with more severe motor disabilities are also more likely to have comorbidities.

These associated comorbidities occur in CP at variable rates. Pain is noted in 75% of CP subjects, intellectual disability in half of them, whereas inability to walk or hip displacement is equally seen in a third. Twenty-five percent of children with CP cannot talk, and a similar proportion carries a diagnosis of epilepsy. Behavioral disorders and urinary incontinence are equally seen in roughly 25% of subjects and sleep disorders in 20%; tube feeding is needed in little less than 10%. Blindness is noted in 10% of cases, with deafness being less common at a rate of 5%.

6. Neuroimaging in cerebral palsy

Head CT scan commonly identifies abnormalities, particularly in spastic CP. Cerebral atrophy is a frequent finding in quadriplegia, whereas infarction, porencephalic cyst, and cerebral atrophy occur equally (26.7%) in hemiplegic CP, and periventricular leukomalacia is significantly more common with diplegia. A brain abnormality seen on CT scan has been reported in 77% of the cases of hemiplegia, followed by quadriplegia (75%) and diplegia (55%) [11], while other studies showed CT abnormalities in 77.2% of patients, with bilateral atrophy in 42.1% and focal findings in 17.6% of the cases [12].

MRI scan is an important and safe diagnostic tool to use in children with CP after 18 months in order to assess location, nature, and structure of brain lesion and correlate findings with clinical picture.

The patterns of MRI in children with cerebral palsy are as follows:

- White matter damage, observed more often in spastic diplegia and quadriplegia.

- Gray matter damage: central gray matter damage of acute perinatal hypoxia-ischemia in term infants is associated with death and CP.

- Enlarged ventricles, bilateral or unilateral, abnormalities of the atria and ventricular or occipital horns, and posterior fossa, atrophy, and cerebrospinal fluid abnormalities [13].

In a European cerebral palsy study [14], MRI was performed in 351 of the 431 children with clinically assessed CP. The MRI scans showed that white matter damage of immaturity, including periventricular leukomalacia, was the most common finding (42.5%, majority born before 34 weeks), followed by basal ganglia lesions (12.8%), cortical/subcortical lesions (9.4%), malformations (9.1%), focal infarcts (7.4%), and miscellaneous lesions (7.1%). Normal MRI findings were present in 11.7%.

MRI scan does provide useful information on the timing and extent of the lesion. Predisposing risk factors include maternal and child genetic factors in thrombophilia leading to stroke, nutritional factors, and infections during

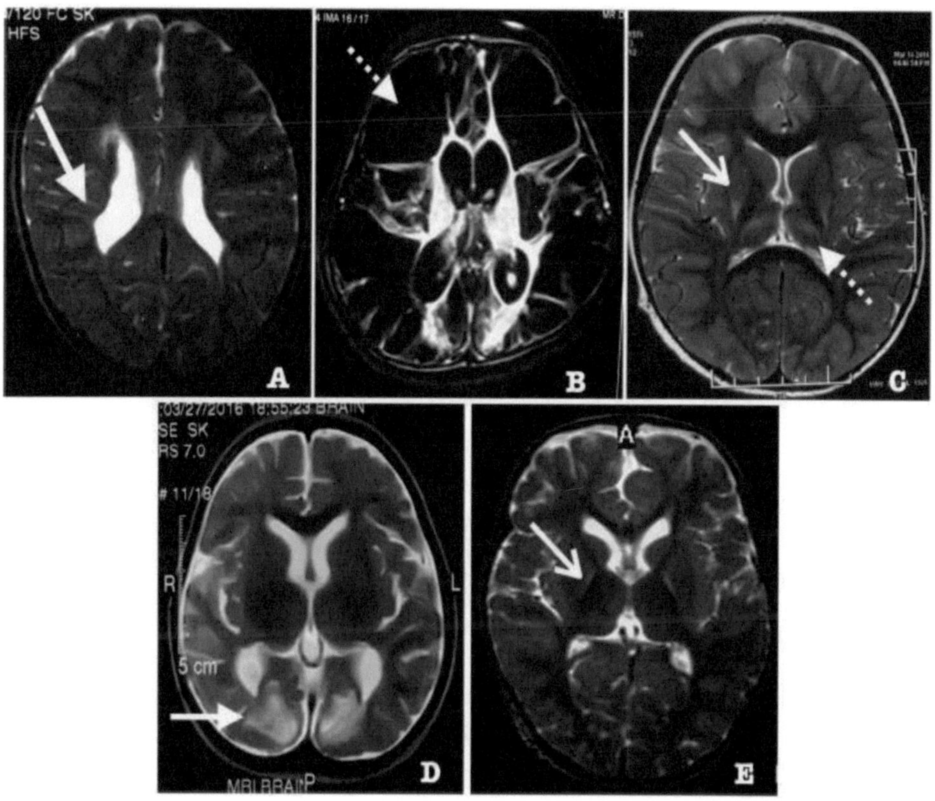

Figure 1.
Salient MRI changes in cerebral palsy. Panel A shows a T2-weighted image with periventricular hyperintensities and undulating ventricular margins (solid arrow). This is typically seen in prematurity associated insult and commonly manifests as spastic diplegia. Panel B shows multicystic encephalomalacia (dotted line with arrow). This pattern of watershed lesions is seen commonly in term infants with ischemia/ asphyxia and manifests clinically with spastic quadriplegia. Panel C illustrates T2 hyperintensities in posterior putamen (open arrow) and thalami bilaterally (dotted line with closed arrow). This is typically seen in infants with term hypoxic ischemic encephalopathy (HIE) and manifests as dyskinetic cerebral palsy. Panel D highlights T2 hyperintensities in occipital lobe (solid arrow); characteristic of neonatal hypoglycemic insult. Panel E shows T2 hyperintensity involving bilateral globuspallidi (open arrow), a feature of kernicterus sequelae.

pregnancy and before the onset of premature labor lead to placental damage developing throughout the pregnancy. These factors predispose the infant to an increased risk of hypoxic ischemic episodes, leading to white matter damage.

It is not unreasonable, therefore, to assume that with increased awareness of possible preventive measures, CP could be reduced substantially, reducing as a consequence the burden on families and saving tremendous sums of money for health services. **Figure 1** shows the MRI findings in CP.

7. Evaluation of patient with cerebral palsy

The diagnostic evaluation must include standardized assessment of neurologic and motor development and magnetic resonance imaging (MRI).

Screening for thrombophilia is recommended in children with MRI evidence of cerebral infarction.

Other testing depends on clinical and anamnestic concerns and may include:

- Metabolic and genetic testing, which should be pursued in the presence of atypical symptoms or MRI findings (e.g., a brain malformation or injury) or if no etiology is identified by clinical history and neuroimaging

- Electroencephalogram (EEG) if seizure activity is suspected

- Infectious work-up (TORCH titers) if pre- or perinatal history is suggestive

All children with CP need to be screened for commonly associated conditions, such as intellectual disability, ophthalmologic abnormalities, hearing impairment, speech and language disorders, and growth failure.

8. Diagnosis of cerebral palsy

A combination of clinical findings supports the diagnosis of CP; a single clinical finding is generally not sufficient to establish the diagnosis.

Key features in the diagnosis of CP include:

1. Abnormal motor development and posture.

2. Brain injury is permanent and nonprogressive.

3. Motor impairment is attributed to an insult that occurred in the developing fetal or infant brain.

4. Motor impairment results in limitations in functional abilities and activities.

5. Motor impairment is often accompanied by secondary musculoskeletal problems, epilepsy, and/or disturbances of sensation, perception, cognition, communication, and behavior.

9. Prognosis of cerebral palsy

Survival to adulthood is currently a standard for most children. An analysis of children with CP born in different geographical areas of the United Kingdom between 1980 and 1996 revealed a 20-year survival in 87–94% of cases [15]. The multivariate analysis revealed that survival was related to severity of impairment, birth weight, and socioeconomic status, with the number of severe impairments having the greatest effect.

Those children who do not achieve head balance by 20 months retain primitive reflexes, have no postural reactions by 24 months, or do not crawl by approximately 5 years of age have generally poor prognosis for walking. Generally, all children with hemiplegic CP and many with athetosis or ataxia will walk. Those who walk independently do so around the age of 3; those who walk only with support may take up to 9 years. Those who do not walk by 9 years of age are unlikely to ever walk, even with support [16].

Functional outcome in CP also depends on other non-motor factors. These include intelligence, physical function, ability to communicate, and personality attributes.

10. Seizures in cerebral palsy patients

Besides the motor dysfunction, epilepsy is another important problem in children with CP. It is sometimes more disabling than the motor disorder itself.

10.1 Incidence of seizures and epilepsy in CP

Epilepsy is highly correlated with CP.

The incidence of epilepsy in CP varies from 33 to 41% [11, 12]. The incidence and type of epilepsy vary according to the type of CP.

The large variation in percentages reported in the literature can be explained in part by the variable length of follow-up periods and the different average age of studied subjects.

Reported rates of seizures and epilepsy in CP vary significantly depending on the underlying pathology and etiology. Epilepsy occurs in 50–94% of children with CP due to diffuse cortical malformations and injuries [17, 18] and in 50% of children with CP secondary to suspected perinatal arterial ischemic stroke [19, 20]. Epilepsy occurs at a much lower frequency (26–43%) in CP and white matter injury (WMI) than in other etiologies [21–24]. The lower frequency of epilepsy and WMI is related to the lack of involvement of cortical gray matter. A recent publication [25] indicated that 25% of children with CP and WMI had seizures beyond the neonatal period with electroclinical features of the age-limited, epileptic syndromes of childhood, with favorable outcome in the majority. Very interesting findings that need to be confirmed, guiding toward better diagnostic, treatment, prognostic, and genetic issues at this early age group.

Seizure onset often occurs in the first 2 years of life. Sixty-one percent of patients with CP had their seizure onset that early. Some reports indicate 36.7% [12] to 69.7% [23] of patients with seizure onset in the first year of life. The onset of epilepsy probably reflects the time of occurrence of brain damage and its severity.

The age of seizure onset also depends on the type of CP. Over 60% of the children with quadriplegia and diplegia have seizures in their first year of life, while 60% of the children with hemiplegia had their first seizure at a later age. Children with myoclonic seizures and infantile spasms had seizure onset very early in life [11].

10.2 Risk factors for seizures in patients with CP

Family history, structural abnormalities (primarily brain atrophy and gray matter involvement), neonatal seizure, low Apgar scores, and mental retardation are significant risk factors for the development of epilepsy in patients with CP.

CP patients with spastic quadriplegia or acquired hemiplegia are more prone to seizures, whereas seizures are less common in mild symmetric spastic diplegia and CP that is mainly athetoid.

The mode of delivery, the relative birth weight, head circumferences, and the presence of consanguinity are not known to be risk factors for epilepsy in these patients.

Risk factors for the development of epilepsy are shown in **Table 2**.

In a study of 452 patients with CP and 160 patients with both CP and epilepsy [11], the incidence of epilepsy among patients with hemiparetic CP was 65.9%, compared to 42.6% in patients with quadriparetic CP and 15.8% in patients with paraparetic CP. The different levels and degrees of brain damage may account for the various percentages.

Other studies revealed that epilepsy was found in 54% of quadriparetic, 34–60% of hemiparetic, 27% of diparetic, and 23–26% of dystonic CP patients [26, 27].

The age at onset of seizures might differ depending on the type of CP. Carlsson et al. reported the seizure onset of age as 6 months in quadriparetic CP, 12 months in diparetic CP, and 2.5 years in hemiparetic CP [21].

10.2.1 Neonatal seizures

Neonatal seizures represent a strong predictor for the development of epilepsy. A strong association of neonatal seizures with epilepsy was reported in the Collaborative Perinatal Project (NCPP) of the NIH summarizing 54,000 singleton pregnancies between 1959 and 1966 [28]. Subsequently, additional retrospective studies provided clear evidence that in children with CP neonatal seizures were strongly predictive for future development of epilepsy [11, 29].

Neonatal seizure history in patients with CP is a risk factor for epilepsy development. In addition, the outcome for seizure control was negatively affected by this history, and patients with neonatal seizure history are 3.3 times more likely to have poor epilepsy prognosis than those who had no neonatal seizure history [30].

	CP With Epilepsy n = 62	CP Without Epilepsy n = 38	
Girl/boy	29/33	19/19	Ns
Neonatal seizures	30	3	p < 0.004
Positive family history	18	1	P < 0.02
CT scan abnormalities	48/57*	15/27**	Ns

Ns, not significant; *48 of 57 patients with CP and epilepsy showed computed tomographic scan abnormalities; **15 of 27 patients with CP and without epilepsy showed computed tomographic scan abnormalities.

Table 2.
Type of CP as a risk factor for seizures.

Hence, neonatal seizure history in CP is a significant risk factor for both epilepsy development and poor epilepsy prognosis.

10.2.2 Family history of epilepsy

Family history of epilepsy is associated with a 5.5 times higher risk of epilepsy in patients with CP [31].

10.2.3 Mental retardation

Mental retardation is more frequently observed in CP patients with seizures than in those without seizures, and severe mental retardation is more likely in those with multiple seizure types.

In patients with CP and mental retardation, the diagnosis of epilepsy presents unique challenges. Generally, patients are unable to describe the epileptic events themselves, parents may not recognize subtle seizure manifestations, and persons trained in epilepsy witness the events only rarely.

Mental retardation is frequently observed in patients with both CP and epilepsy compared to patients with CP only. In addition, the risk of epilepsy development is higher in patients with CP who have mental retardation [32, 33].

Patients with CP and epilepsy have lower intelligence levels compared with CP alone; the patients with paroxysmal abnormalities in the EEG had lower intelligence levels and learning disabilities [34].

Mental retardation is most common in quadriplegic CP, followed by hemiplegic CP. On the contrary, almost half of diplegic CP and 60% of children with dystonic CP have normal to borderline intelligence, which again correlates well with the type and location of brain damage. Mental retardation is associated with earlier age of onset, increased frequency, and treatment-resistant seizures [11]. This might represent an underlying severity of brain injury that is responsible for the severity of both cognitive deficit and epilepsy.

10.2.4 Apgar score and risk of seizures in CP patients

The risk of epilepsy is inversely proportional to the Apgar scores of term babies, both at 5 and 10 minutes. This is significant even with relatively minor reductions in these scores [35].

Low Apgar scores were also recognized as risk factors for epilepsy in the general population in some other studies [36, 37].

No relationship has been found between the risk of epilepsy development and gestational age [31]. In a study where 173 patients were categorized according to their birth weight as appropriate for gestational age (76.9%), small for gestational age (12.1%), and large for gestational age (11%), they found no correlation between birth weight and risk of epilepsy development [38].

However, other studies reveal that low birth weight and prematurity increase the risk of epilepsy development in patients with CP [12, 37, 39]. These studies assessed Apgar scores and determined that premature babies have lower Apgar scores; they suggested that the increased risk of epilepsy development among premature babies was actually related to low Apgar scores.

10.3 Types of seizures

All types of epileptic seizures can be seen in patients with CP. Focal impaired awareness (complex partial) and focal to generalized tonic-clonic are the most

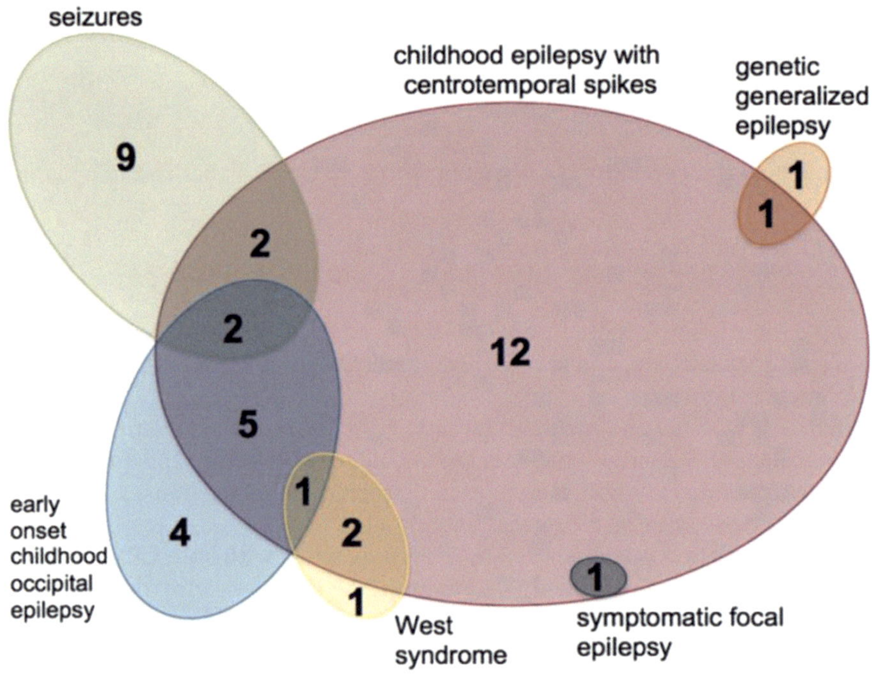

Figure 2.
Epileptic syndromes in 41 children with cerebral palsy.

Seizure Type	SPQ (n = 53)	SPD (n = 20)	SPH (n = 22)	DYS (n = 5)	HYPO (n = 3)	Mixed (n = 2)	Overall (n = 105)
GTC	19 (35.1%)	9 (45%)	7 (31.8%)	1 (20%)	3 (100%)	1 (50%)	40 (38.1%)
SP	3 (5.7%)	3 (15%)	1 (4.5%)	1 (20%)	0	1 (50%)	9 (8.6%)
CP	6 (11.3%)	1 (5%)	6 (27.3%)	0	0	0	13 (12.4%)
P-SG	7 (13.2%)	3 (15%)	3 (13.6%)	0	0	0	13 (12.4%)
MJ	9 (17%)	3 (15%)	1 (4.5%)	2 (40%)	0	0	15 (14.3%)
IS	14 (26.4%)	5 (25%)	3 (13.6%)	1 (20%)	0	0	23 (22%)
Others	0	1 (5%)	0	0	0	0	1 (1%)

CP = complex partial; DYS = dyskinetic; GTC = generalized tonic clonic; HYPO = hypotonic; IS = infantile spasms; MJ = myoclonic jerks; P-SG = partial with secondary generalization; SP = simple partial; SPD = spastic diplegia; SPH = spastic hemiplegia; SPQ = spastic quadriplegia.

Table 3.
Types of seizures in subtypes of CP [11].

frequent seizure types. Some syndromes, such as infantile spasms, West, and Lennox-Gastaut syndromes, are particularly frequent.

Generalized epilepsy is the predominant form of epilepsy in CP. Generalized seizures have been reported in 36.8%, followed by focal (partial) seizures in 33%, West syndrome in 15.6%, and myoclonic jerks in 10.6%. Absence seizures are usually of the atypical type reported in 3.3–6.7% [3].

In another study of patients with both CP and epilepsy, the following seizure types were observed: 44.6% experience focal to generalized tonic-clonic, 41.1%

focal impaired awareness (complex partial), 7.1% focal aware (simple partial), 5.4% myoclonic, and 1.8% experience atonic seizures [30]. This finding is in line with the literature review [31]. **Figure 2** and **Table 3** show epileptic syndromes and types of seizures in subtypes of CP in children with cerebral palsy.

10.4 Electroencephalogram (EEG)

EEG is essential in the work-up of children with CP and suspected seizures. It can lend support to the diagnosis of epilepsy and assist in seizure/epilepsy classification to better guide the choice of antiseizure drugs. However, there is no clinical value of performing EEG testing in children with no suggestion of seizure activity by history, and EEG testing is not useful in establishing the cause of CP.

The rate of EEG abnormalities observed in patients with CP and epilepsy is in the range of 66–92.6% [4, 11, 31].

All of the subgroups of spastic CP had a greater than 70% incidence of abnormal EEGs. Whereas in quadriplegic and diplegic CP, the EEG shows predominant bilateral epileptic activity; about half of children with hemiplegia had focal findings. In a study of children with CP and epilepsy, only 7.9% of children had normal interictal EEGs [**Table 4**] [4].

There was a correlation between brain CT scan and EEG findings; children with bilateral brain abnormalities on their CT scan imaging often had bilateral and generalized epileptiform abnormalities on their EEGs. However, one-fourth of these children had a focal epileptiform abnormality with rapid bilateral synchrony. On the other hand, 35.3% of children with unilateral structural brain abnormalities on their CT scans had focal epileptiform abnormalities in their EEG recordings; the EEG findings were concordant with the CT scan findings in all patients [11].

10.5 Neuroimaging in cerebral palsy with epilepsy

Children with CP and epilepsy appear to have abnormal brain imaging more often. It is not surprising that a trend toward the occurrence of epilepsy was found in children with gray matter insult (primarily cerebral infarcts), rather than in children with white matter lesions. In addition, cerebral atrophy was also reported more frequently in CP complicated by epilepsy [31], reaching statistical significance in the study of Gururaj et al. [40]. A possible explanation for the association of

EEG	SPQ (n = 53)	SPD (n = 20)	SPH (n = 22)	DYS (n = 5)	HYPO (n = 3)	Mixed (n = 2)	Total (n = 105)
Generalized activity	21	10	9	2	2	0	44
Focal activity	5	2	4	2	0	0	13
Focal onset—bilateral synchrony	10	3	3	0	0	1	7
Total	36 (67.9%)	15 (75%)	16 (72.7%)	4 (80%)	2 (66.6%)	1 (50%)	74 (70.5%)

DYS = dyskinetic; HYPO = hypotonic; SPD = spastic diplegia; SPH = spastic hemiplegia; SPQ = spastic quadriplegia.

Table 4.
EEG abnormality and type of CP.

Imaging findings	CP Only	CP & Epilepsy	Total
Normal imaging	25 (28.7%)	10 (16.4%)	35 (23.6%)
Abnormal Imaging (all findings)	62 (71.3%)	51 (83.6%)	113 (76.4%)
Non-specific atrophy	4 (4.6 %)	11 (18.0%)	16 (10.8%)
Grey matter insult (including infarctions)	14 (16.1%)	17 (27.9%)	31 (21.0%)
White matter insult (including PVL)	16 (18.4%)	4 (11.5%)	23 (15.5%)
Cerebral malformations Dysgenesis	10 (11.5%)	7 (11.5%)	17 (11.5%)
Hydrocephalus	5 (5.7%)	5 (8.2%)	8 (5.4%)
Brain Hemorrhage (including IVH)	13 (14.9%)	7 (11.5%)	20 (13.5%)
Total	87 (100%)	61 (100%)	148 (100%)

Abbreviations: PVL - Periventricular Leukomalacia, and IVH - Intraventricular Hemorrhage.
$p < 0.003$.

Table 5.
Imaging findings in patients with cerebral palsy only and with cerebral palsy and epilepsy.

atrophy and epilepsy is the fact that in many cases atrophy presents the end result of prenatal or perinatal global ischemia with extensive neuronal damage.

Intraventricular hemorrhage was identified as a significant risk factor for the development of neonatal seizures [41]. In patients with neonatal seizures, cerebral dysgenesis and intraventricular hemorrhage proved to be predictors for poor outcome [29].

Brain imaging in children with CP and epilepsy shows frequently abnormal findings. In children with CP and epilepsy, cerebral atrophy is more often reported [31, 40]. Atrophy is the consequence of prenatal and perinatal ischemia; this will lead to an extensive neuronal damage which may be the cause of the seizures. A significant risk factor for the development of neonatal seizures was found with intraventricular hemorrhage [41]. Cerebral dysgenesis and intraventricular hemorrhage were found to be predictors of poor outcome in patients with neonatal seizures [29].

The effect of imaging abnormalities in CP remains controversial. In one study, an MRI abnormality was noted in 86.7% of patients, and the abnormal finding variable in the MRI did not significantly affect the epilepsy development and seizure outcome.

In other studies the range of abnormal findings in MRI was reported as 84–88% [42]. Cerebral infarct is found by neuroimaging to be an abnormality that significantly affects seizure outcome in epileptic patients with CP [4]. **Table 5** shows the imaging findings in patients with CP and epilepsy and CP without epilepsy.

10.6 Seizure control

More than 50% of seizures in patients with CP are fairly controlled. Seizures in patients with hemiplegic CP achieve better control (75%) than those with quadriplegic and diplegic CP (50%); one study reported seizure control in children with CP in nearly two-thirds [4]. Seizure control was achieved with monotherapy in the majority of cases. Polytherapy was required in half, one-third, and one-fourth of cases with diplegic, quadriplegic, and hemiplegic CP, respectively, although this difference did not reach statistical significance. In another study by Hadjipanayis et al., children with spastic hemiplegia (35%) and tetraplegia (28%) were more likely to require polytherapy compared to patients with spastic diplegia (11%) [3]; however, the differences were not statistically significant [3]. Not surprising, polytherapy was required more often in children with infantile spasms and myoclonic seizures. All other seizure characteristics also were more severe in the group requiring polytherapy. In addition, a trend was noted for the following: seizures began earlier, and CT and EEG abnormalities were more often present in children requiring polytherapy.

10.7 Cerebral palsy: recommendation and future directions

The rate of CP has remained static for decades, at between 2 and 2.5 cases for every 1000 live births, due to abnormalities of the developing fetal or infantile brain resulting from a variety of causes. In a recent publication, however, Hollung et al. reported that the prevalence of CP declined for children born in Norway from 2.62 per 1000 in 1999 to 1.89 in 2010, and in addition a substantial improvement in the severity of clinical characteristics with a decrease in the proportion of children with severe motor impairments, epilepsy, intellectual disability, and difficult to understand or no speech was observed. They attributed this improvement to the better obstetric and neonatal care the first decade of the twenty-first century [43]. In general, however, methods that have been implemented, such as continuous electronic monitoring of the fetus in labor, have not had the anticipated benefits. Many neuroprotective strategies have failed. In premature infants, an increase in survival without a decrease in prevalence added more healthy citizens but also more disabled children to the population. As a consequence in recent years, efforts have focused on prevention, cure, early diagnosis, and early intervention in an attempt to reduce further CP prevalence.

Approximately one-half of all new cases of cerebral palsy arise from the group of neonates born prematurely (< 30 weeks gestation) that are at risk for long-term neurodevelopmental problems, with almost one-half having motor, cognitive, and/or language impairments, a rate much higher than their term peers [44]. For many children, however, the cause of cerebral palsy is unclear. There are many known risk factors that affect the fetal and neonatal developing brain leading to cerebral palsy, and some of them can be prevented. Risk factors for congenital CP include infection during pregnancy (toxoplasmosis, rubella, cytomegalovirus, and herpes can infect the womb and placenta, leading to brain damage in the fetus), abuses of alcohol or drugs during pregnancy, smoking, exposure to toxic chemicals, multiple gestations, and infertility treatments that have an increased risk in preterm delivery and multiple gestations and certain medical conditions such as diabetes, high blood pressure, abnormal thyroid function, sexually transmitted infections, and eating disorders (anorexia nervosa, bulimia nervosa, binge eating disorder). Placental infarctions are most likely to be identified in the births of infants who will in the future develop cerebral palsy, especially those with spastic quadriplegia, an early reliable biomarker.

Before pregnancy we have to make sure that the woman is protected against certain diseases such as rubella with vaccination and certain preventable infections or cytomegalovirus (CMV). CMV in particular, is transmitted through close person-to-person contact with infected secretions such as in urine and saliva. The infection is transmitted from the mother to the fetus during pregnancy and can sometimes cause stillbirth, premature birth, and neurological conditions such as cerebral palsy. Children with cerebral palsy infected with CMV are more likely to have spastic quadriplegia, severe functional mobility limitations and a range of associated impairments including epilepsy, deafness, vision impairment, and moderate-to-severe intellectual disabilities, than children born with cerebral palsy but without CMV. There is evidence that public health approaches based on hygiene can dramatically reduce the rate of primary maternal cytomegalovirus infections during pregnancy. Formulated consensus recommendations on the diagnosis, prevention, and treatment of maternal and congenital CMV infection are found in the publication of Rawlinson et al. [45].

Our primary aim, therefore, is to provide a healthy pregnancy by advising and treating appropriately treatable conditions and introduce current preventable strategies and interventions that hold promise for reducing the prevalence of cerebral palsy. Such interventions include strategies to decrease the risk of premature birth (e.g., 17α-progesterone), limit the number of multiple gestations related to assisted reproductive technology, treat mothers who are expected to deliver prior to 30 weeks gestation with magnesium sulfate for fetal neuroprotection that can prevent cerebral palsy, give antenatal steroids for mothers expected to deliver prematurely, caffeine for extremely low-birth-weight neonates, and induce hypothermia for a subgroup of neonates diagnosed with intrapartum hypoxic-ischemic encephalopathy [46]. Hypothermia, either selectively applied to the head or total body, appears to decrease the risk of cerebral palsy [47]. Interventions which either prolong gestation or decrease the risk of preterm delivery will also decrease the risk of cerebral palsy.

Although ~50% of very preterm children has neurodevelopmental impairments, an early prediction of infants who will experience problems later in life still remains an early diagnostic challenge. White matter abnormalities (WMA) at term have been associated with CP in very preterm children and can be used as a biomarker for early multidisciplinary approach. Very preterm children with any WMA at term require follow-up throughout childhood [48]. Abnormal general movements in very preterm infants born <30 weeks gestation, particularly at 3 months post term, are predictive of worse neurodevelopment at ages 2 and 4 years and need multidisciplinary approach. The accuracy for predicting moderate to severe cognitive impairment was good at 83% and 77% for 2 and 4 years, respectively [49].

Recent research on neuroplasticity supports intensive, repetitive, task-specific intervention for CP that should commence early while the brain is most plastic. Early postnatal recognition is important for a prompt referral to diagnostic-specific early intervention setting to optimize infant's motor and cognitive plasticity, prevent secondary complications, and enhance caregiver's well-being [50].

Beside traditional conventional therapies, physical therapy, occupational therapy, and speech-language therapy, a number of other approaches have been used such as the use of Botox, selective dorsal rhizotomy, functional vision assessment and intervention programs, developmental optometry, biofeedback, hippotherapy, hyperbaric oxygen therapy, deep brain stimulation for dyskinetic forms of cerebral palsy, stem cell applications, and even yoga. It is very difficult to decide which method is "gold standard" type of therapy for CP because it is impossible to conduct double-blind, randomized control trials. However, identifying predictive biomarkers and developing preventive strategies phenotypically orientated to different subsyndromes, we can prevent or intervene early taking into consideration the advantage of brain plasticity.

11. Conclusions

In general children with CP have epileptic seizures in about one-third that occur as a rule within the first 2 years of life. The most common seizure type is focal generalized seizures followed by focal, infantile spasms, and myoclonic seizures that are seen in one-fourth of cases. Seizures are most often seen in spastic hemiplegia and spastic quadriplegia. Children with CP and mental retardation have an early onset of seizures and more severe epilepsy. The response to antiseizure treatment in children with CP is generally difficult, and one-third to half of the cases is receiving polytherapy and/or alternative therapies.

Author details

Boulenouar Mesraoua[1,2*], Musab Ali[1], Dirk Deleu[1,2], Hassan Al Hail[1,2], Gayane Melikyan[1,2], Naim Haddad[2], Osama Alalamy[1,2], Covanis Athanasios[3] and Ali A. Asadi-Pooya[4,5]

1 Hamad Medical Corporation, Doha, Qatar

2 Weill Cornell Medical College, Doha, Qatar

3 Neurology and Neurophysiology Department, The Children's Hospital Agia Sophia, Athens, Greece

4 Department of Neurology, Thomas Jefferson University, Philadelphia, PA, USA

5 Department of Neurology, Shiraz University of Medical Sciences, Shiraz, Iran

*Address all correspondence to: boulenouar.mesraoua@wanadoo.fr

References

[1] Mutch L, Alberman E, Hagberg B, et al. Cerebral palsy epidemiology: Where are we now and where are we going? Developmental Medicine & Child Neurology. 1992;**34**:547-551

[2] The definition and classification of cerebral palsy. Developmental Medicine and Child Neurology. 2007;**49**:1-44

[3] Hadjipanayis A, Hadjichristodoulou C, Youroukos S. Epilepsy in patients with cerebral palsy. Developmental Medicine and Child Neurology. 1997;**39**: 659-663

[4] Zafeiriou D, Eleftherios E, Kontopoulos E, Tsikoulas I. Characteristics and prognosis of epilepsy in children with cerebral palsy. Journal of Child Neurology. 1999;**14**: 289-294

[5] Oskoui M, Coutinho F, Dykeman J, et al. An update on the prevalence of cerebral palsy: A systematic review and meta-analysis. Developmental Medicine and Child Neurology. 2013;**55**:509

[6] Hirvonen M, Ojala R, Korhonen P, et al. Cerebral palsy among children born moderately and late preterm. Pediatrics. 2014;**134**:e1584

[7] Pharoah PO, Platt MJ, Cooke T. The changing epidemiology of cerebral palsy. Archives of Disease in Childhood. Fetal and Neonatal Edition. 1996;**75**: F169

[8] Platt MJ, Cans C, Johnson A, et al. Trends in cerebral palsy among infants of very low birthweight (<1500 g) or born prematurely (<32 weeks) in 16 European centres: A database study. Lancet. 2007;**369**:43

[9] Strijbis EM, Oudman I, van Essen P, MacLennan AH. Cerebral palsy and the application of the international criteria for acute intrapartum hypoxia. Obstetrics & Gynecology. 2006, 107: 1357

[10] Venter A, Schirm N, Joubert G, Fock J. Profile of children diagnosed with cerebral palsy at universitas hospital, Bloemfontein, 1991–2001. South African Family Practice. 2006;**48**: 15. Available from: http://www.tandfonline.com/doi/abs/10.1080/20786204.2006.1087335

[11] Novak I, Hines M, Goldsmith S, Barclay R. Clinical prognostic messages from a systematic review on cerebral palsy. Pediatrics. 2012;**130**(5):e1285-e1312

[12] Singhi P, Jagirdar S, Khandelwal N, Malhi P. Epilepsy in children with cerebral palsy. Journal of Child Neurology. 2003;**18**:174e9

[13] Pedersen H, Taudorf K, Melchior JC. Computed tomography in spastic cerebral palsy. Neuroradiology. 1982;**23**:275-278

[14] Aksu F. Nature and prognosis of seizures in patients with cerebral palsy. Developmental Medicine and Child Neurology. 1990;**32**:661-668

[15] Bjorgaas H, Elgen I, Boe T, Hysing M. Mental health in children with cerebral palsy: Does screening capture the complexity? Hindawi publishing corporation. The Scientific World Journal. 2013;**4**:1-8

[16] Mirmiran M, Barnes P, Keller K, Constantinou J, Fleisher B, Hintz S, et al. Magnetic resonance imaging findings in a population-based cohort of children with cerebral palsy. The Journal of Pediatrics. 2004;**114**(4):992-998

[17] Bax M, Tydeman C, Flodmark O. Clinical and MRI correlates of cerebral palsy. The European cerebral palsy study. JAMA. 2006;**296**(13):1602-1608

[18] Rosenbaum P, Paneth N, Leviton A, et al. A report: The definition and classification of cerebral palsy April 2006. Developmental Medicine and Child Neurology. Supplement. 2007; **109**:8

[19] Hemming K, Hutton JL, Colver A, Platt MJ. Regional variation in survival of people with cerebral palsy in the United Kingdom. Pediatrics. 2005;**116**: 1383-1390

[20] da Paz Junior AC, Burnett SM, Braga LW. Walking prognosis in cerebral palsy: A 22-year retrospective analysis. Developmental Medicine and Child Neurology. 1994;**36**:130-134

[21] Reid SM, Dagia CD, Ditchfield MR, Reddihough DS. Grey matter injury patterns in cerebral palsy: Associations between structural involvement on MRI and clinical outcomes. Developmental Medicine and Child Neurology. 2015; **57**(12):1159-1167

[22] Carlsson M, Hagberg G, Olsson I. Clinical and aetiological aspects of epilepsy in children with cerebral palsy. Developmental Medicine and Child Neurology. 2003;**45**(6):371-376

[23] Wanigasinghe J, Reid SM, Mackay MT, Reddihough DS, Harvey AS, Freeman JL. Epilepsy in hemiplegic cerebral palsy due to perinatal arterial ischaemic stroke. Developmental Medicine and Child Neurology. 2010; **52**(11):1021-1027

[24] Fukuda K, Kirino T, Fujiwara Y, Nagai S, Endo S. Clinical aspects of epilepsy in children with periventricular leukomalacia [in Japanese]. No to Hattatsu. 2010;**42**(4):291-295

[25] Cooper MS, Mackay MT, Fahey M, Reddihough D, Reid SM, Williams K, et al. Seizures in children with cerebral palsy and white matter injury. Pediatrics. 2017;**139**(3):e20162975

[26] Aicardi J. Epilepsy in brain injured children. Developmental Medicine and Child Neurology. 1990;**32**:191e202

[27] Jacobs IB. Epilepsy. In: Thompson GH, Rubin IL, Bilenker RM, editors. Comprehensive Management of Cerebral Palsy. New York: Grune and Tratton; 1983. p. 131e7

[28] Nelson KB, Ellenberg JH. Antecedents of seizure disorders in early childhood. American Journal of Diseases of Children. 1986;**140**:1053-1061

[29] Ronen GM, Buckley D, Penney S, Streiner DL. Long-term prognosis in children with neonatal seizures: A populationbased study. Neurology. 2007;**69**:1816-1822

[30] Mert GG, Incecik F, Altunbasak S, Herguner O, Mert MK, Kiris N, et al. Factors affecting epilepsy development and epilepsy prognosis in cerebral palsy. Pediatric Neurology. 2011;**45**(2):89-94

[31] Kulak W, Sobaniec W. Risk factors and prognosis of epilepsy in children with cerebral palsy in North-Eastern Poland. Brain Development. 2003;**27**: 499e506

[32] Goulden KJ, Shinnar S, Koller H. Epilepsy in children with mental retardation: A chart study. Epilepsia. 1991;**32**:690e7

[33] Steffenberg U, Hagberg G, Kyllerman M. Characteristics of seizures in a population- based series of mentally retarded children with active epilepsy. Epilepsia. 1996;**37**:850e6

[34] Wallace SJ. Epilepsy in cerebral palsy. Developmental Medicine and Child Neurology. 2001;**43**:713e7

[35] Persson M, Razaz N, Tedroff K, Joseph KS, Cnattingius S. Five and 10 minute Apgar scores and risks of cerebral palsy and epilepsy: Population

based cohort study in Sweden. BMJ. 2018;**360**:k207

[36] Sun Y, Vestergaard M, Pedersen CB, Christensen J, Olsen J. Apgar scores and long-term risk of epilepsy. Epidemiology. 2006;**17**:296-301

[37] Ehrenstein V, Sørensen HT, Pedersen L, Larsen H, Holsteen V, Rothman KJ. Apgar score and hospitalization for epilepsy in childhood: A registry-based cohort study. BMC Public Health. 2006;**6**:23

[38] Zelnik N, Konopnicki M, Bennett-Back O, Castel-Dutch T, Tirosh E. Risk factors for epilepsy in children with cerebral palsy. European Journal of Paediatric Neurology. 2009;**30**:1e6

[39] Odding E, Roebroeck ME, Stam HJ. The epidemiology of cerebral palsy: Incidence, impairments and risk factors. Disability and Rehabilitation. 2006;**28**: 183e91

[40] Gururaj AK, Sztriha L, Bener A, Dawadou A, Eapen V. Epilepsy in children with cerebral palsy. Seizure. 2003;**12**:110e4

[41] Kohelet D, Shochat R, Lusky A, Reichman B. Israel neonatal network. Risk factors for seizures in very low birthweight infants with periventricular leukomalacia. Journal of Child Neurology. 2006;**21**:965-970

[42] Robinson MN, Peake JL, Ditchfield MR, Reid MS, Lanigan A, Reddihough DS. Magnetic resonance imaging findings in a population based cohort of children with cerebral epilepsy. Developmental Medicine and Child Neurology. 2008;**51**:39e45

[43] Hollung SJ, Vik T, Lydersen S, Bakken IJ, Andersen GL. Decreasing prevalence and severity of cerebral palsy in Norway among children born 1999 to 2010 concomitant with improvements in perinatal health. European Journal of Paediatric Neurology. 2018;**22**:814-821

[44] Saigal S, Doyle LW. An overview of mortality and sequelae of preterm birth from infancy to adulthood. Lancet. 2008;**371**(9608):261-269

[45] Rawlinson WD, Boppana SB, Fowler KB, et al. Congenital cytomegalovirus infection in pregnancy and the neonate: Consensus recommendations for prevention, diagnosis, and therapy. The Lancet Infectious Diseases. 2017;**17**(6): e177-e188

[46] O'Shea TM. Diagnosis, treatment, and prevention of cerebral palsy in near-term/term infants. Clinical Obstetrics and Gynecology. 2008;**51**(4):816-828. DOI: 10.1097/GRF.0b013e3181870ba7

[47] Shankaran S, Laptook AR, Ehrenkranz RA, Tyson JE, McDonald SA, Donovan EF, et al. Whole-body hypothermia for neonates with hypoxic-ischemic encephalopathy. New England Journal of Medicine. 2005;**353**(15): 1574-1584

[48] Spittle AJ, Cheong J, Doyle LW, Roberts G, Lee JK, Lim J, et al. Neonatal white matter abnormality predicts childhood motor impairment in very preterm children. Developmental Medicine and Child Neurology. 2011; **53**(11):1000-1006. DOI: 10.1111/ j.1469-8749.2011.04095.x

[49] Spittle AJ, Spencer-Smith MM, Cheong JL, Eeles AL, et al. General movements in very preterm children and neurodevelopment at 2 and 4 years. Pediatrics. 2013;**132**(12):e452-e458

[50] Novak I, Morgan C, Adde L, Blackman J, Boyd RN, et al. Early, Accurate Diagnosis and Early Intervention in Cerebral Palsy: Advances in Diagnosis and Treatment. JAMA Pediatrics. 2017;**171**(9): 897-907

Chapter 5

The Role of the DNA Damage Response in Ataxia-Telangiectasia Syndrome

Albert Ribes-Zamora

Abstract

The DNA damage response (DDR) is a concerted response involving a myriad of pathways that cells elicit in the presence of DNA injuries. Patients bearing mutations in DDR genes have an increased cancer incidence derived from their diminished ability to respond to DNA damage, and the consequent increase in mutations. Intriguingly, mutations in ATM, the chief DDR regulator, can cause ataxia telangiectasia, a neurodegenerative disorder characterized by progressive loss of movement coordination, weak immune system, and increased cancer risk. The relationship between ATM and neural system development and degeneration remains to be fully elucidated and will be discussed in this chapter.

Keywords: ATM, DNA damage response, ataxia telangiectasia, neurodegeneration

1. Introduction

Mammalian cells face an estimate of 10^5 genomic injuries every day. These lesions are diverse and can include, among others, single (SSB) and double strand breaks (DSB), oxidative damage, DNA inter- and intra-strand crosslinking, base mismatches, bulky adducts, and photoproducts [1, 2]. This large variety of DNA lesions is directly related to the full range of mutation-causing agents that threaten the genome on a daily basis. Some of these agents are endogenously produced by the cell's own metabolism and homeostasis, while others are generated exogenously. The frequency of appearance of these lesions is also diverse, and it may depend on the cell type or the developmental stage [1]. For instance, skin epithelial cells are much more susceptible to photoproducts caused by ultraviolet rays, an exogenous source of mutations that can only reach the outermost layers of our body. In contrast, reactive oxygen species (ROS) are endogenous metabolic byproducts that can induce oxidative base modifications and SSB, one of the most common genomic injuries. Cells with high energy and metabolic demands are, therefore, most susceptible to suffer SSB-related and other ROS-related injuries.

To defend from the menacing threat that this wide range and number of lesions pose to the integrity of their genome, cells can invoke the DNA damage response (DDR), a vast network of overlapping pathways that is capable of tailoring a response depending on the type and extent of the lesion and the cell cycle stage at the moment of the injury [3–6]. DDR requires the coordination of DNA repair pathways with cell cycle progression regulation, transcription activation, and apoptosis, among other pathways [5, 7, 8].

Somewhat surprisingly, mutations in genes belonging to DDR pathways correlate with neurodevelopmental defects and neurodegenerative pathologies [5, 9–11]. For instance, individuals with dysfunctional versions of SSB repair genes APTX, PNPK, or XRCC1 manifest different types of ataxias with ocular apraxia; whereas, defective TDP1, also involved in SSB repair, can cause spinocerebellar ataxia with axonal neuropathy [9, 12]. Similarly, mutations in DSB repair gene MRE11, or central DDR regulators ATM and ATR, can lead to cerebellar ataxia [5, 13]. Besides ataxias, microcephaly is commonly found linked to defects in several DDR associated genes [1, 5, 14]. Mutations in NBS1 and RAD50, two genes involved in end processing during DSB repair, can cause Nijmegen breakage syndrome (NBS) and NBS-like syndrome, respectively, both syndromes manifesting microcephaly among other conditions [5, 15, 16]. Microcephalia is also present in individuals with dysfunctional PNPK, LIG4—a gene involved in DSB repair—or Seckel Syndrome 1, a developmental disorder caused by some ATR mutations [9, 15]. Furthermore, around 25% of patients with defective nucleotide excision repair (NER)—a DDR pathway in charge of healing photoproducts created by UV light exposure—can also present microcephaly among other neurological problems [5]. Overall, this data suggest a strong and intriguing link between DDR, neurodevelopment, and neuropathology. This review focuses on ATM, its role during DDR, and the molecular basis of ataxia-telangiectasia (A-T), a neurodegenerative syndrome caused by defective or absent ATM.

2. ATM roles during DDR

ATM and ATR are two kinases belonging to the protein phosphatidylinositol-3-kinase-like kinases (PIKK) family that function as the chief regulators of DDR [3, 11, 13]. Together, they coordinate all pathways implicated in DDR to offer an adequate and timely response proportionate to the type and extent of the genomic injury. Recently, DNA-PKcs, another member of the PIKK family, has also been found playing more substantial roles in regulating DDR than initially thought, albeit to a lesser extent that ATM and ATR [17].

ATM is a very large kinase of 3056 amino acids and a molecular weight of 350.6 kD that resides in the nucleus as inactive homodimers. Upon DNA damage infliction, phosphorylation of a critical ATM residue disrupts dimerization, prompting monomers to undergo further phosphorylation to achieve full kinase activation [18–20]. Active ATM monomers phosphorylate substrates on serine or threonine residues followed by glutamine (S/TQ), and a significant amount of ATM substrates contain clusters of S/TQ sites in short stretches of the protein [21]. These so-called SCD domains can be used to mine the proteome for putative ATM targets [22–24]. Using mass spectrometry, a high-throughput screen for proteins phosphorylated following DNA damage found 686 putative DDR targets and the final number is estimated to surpass a thousand proteins [25]. These large numbers showcase the complexity of DDR, and the need for an orchestrated coordination of all pathways involved. Some of the most important direct ATM targets are CHK2 and p53, two downstream effectors that modulate pivotal DDR pathways like cell cycle progression regulation, DNA repair, or apoptosis [26–28].

2.1 DNA repair

ATM is not only activated by different kinds of DNA damage but can also actively participate in several DNA repair mechanisms and coordinate their activities with other DDR-related pathways [7, 29]. During DSB repair, ATM plays crucial roles in the early end-processing events, signal amplification, and recruitment of other DNA repair proteins to the sites of damage [3, 13]. ATM functions in homologous recombination (HR) and nonhomologous end-joining (NHEJ), the two pathways entrusted by cells to repair DSBs. Whereas, NHEJ is active throughout the cell cycle, its function is mostly limited to G0/G1 as S/G2 phases prefer the more accurate HR, a mechanism that uses sister chromatids only present during those phases as repair templates. The first sensor of DSBs is PARP1, which in addition to binding breaks, also adds branches of poly-(ADP)-ribose to proteins post-translationally [30]. This so-called PARylation process activates and recruits several DNA repair proteins to the sites of damage [31]. One of them is the MRN complex—made up of MRE11, RAD50, and NBS1—that binds and activates ATM [32, 33]. Interaction with PARP1 and NBS1, thus, activates and recruits ATM to DSB sites, where it phosphorylates several downstream targets and effectors to amplify DDR signaling. For instance, ATM phosphorylates histone variant H2AX, which promotes MDC1 binding to the chromatin surrounding DSB [34–36]. Once there, ATM-mediated phosphorylation of MDC1 promotes its binding to MRN, and recruitment of more ATM to phosphorylate more H2AX, further spreading DDR signaling [13].

Although the complete process remains to be fully elucidated, it is clear that ATM is also involved in the decision-making process that selects either HR or NHEJ to repair a DSB [37, 38]. A crucial step in this process is the extent of end resection that takes place at DSB [39]. ATM directly phosphorylates CtIP and BRCA1, two HR proteins required for resection initiation and binding of RAD51 to ssDNA ends, respectively [40–42]. Once formed, RAD51 coated 3′ ssDNA ends steer repair toward HR by initiating strand invasion into the sister chromatid. Intriguingly, ATM phosphorylates p53BP1 and promotes its recruitment to sites of DNA damage [43]. Phosphorylated p53BP1 has opposing roles to CtIP and BRCA1, and favors the formation of p53BP1 containing complexes at DSB that counteract HR in favor of NHEJ repair [38, 44]. ATM also influences NHEJ by mediating DNA-PKcs phosphorylation and subsequent recruitment of Artemis, an end-processing nuclease, to DSB sites [45].

Although ATM is mostly activated by DSBs, recent data suggest that some lesions that are usually repaired by BER can also activate ATM and that ATM-dependent phosphorylation events can regulate BER [46]. Following base damage, BER requires the sequential action of DNA glycosylases—to remove damaged bases and create apyrimidinic or apurinic (AP) sites, PARP1—to PARylate the AP site, and endonucleases that will generate an SSB at the AP site [47]. These events can lead to ATM activation and the ATM-dependent phosphorylation of CHK2 [46]. Upon activation, CHK2 phosphorylates XRCC1, a BER protein required for sealing the nick and completing the repair.

DDR is capable of modulating DNA repair pathways through multiple effectors. For instance, both ATR and p53 regulate NER through quite distinct mechanisms. While ATR phosphorylates XPA, one of the earliest respondents to pyrimidine photodimers and other bulky lesions, DDR-dependent phosphorylation of p53 acts by upregulating expression of NER genes and recruiting XPC and TFIIH to sites of damage [7, 48–52]. ATR also regulates ICLR through the phosphorylation of several members of the Fanconi anemia group, a set of proteins that in combination with NER and HR, repair DNA cross-linkage damage [53–55]. Other examples of DDR-signaling-dependent regulation of DNA repair mechanisms include the upregulation of BER through the stimulatory binding of p53 to BER proteins, the promotion of HR that ensues after disruption of the p53-RPA complex by ATM, ATR and DNA-PKcs phosphorylation, and the PIKK-dependent phosphorylation of Werner syndrome and Bloom syndrome proteins involved in DSB repair [56–60].

2.2 Cell cycle progression regulation

One of the most dangerous threats of DNA damage is the possibility of spreading to daughter cells during cell duplication. To prevent this, DDR is capable of halting cell cycle progression at any point during the cell cycle [61]. A series of overlapping mechanisms ensure that cells attempt DNA repair before progressing to the next cell cycle stage [7].

ATM is in charge of preventing lesions produced during G1/G0 to enter S phase, which is particularly important for some of the most common DNA injuries like oxidative damage. Since G1/G0 duration is usually longer than other cell cycle phases, exposure to ROS and other mutating agents is also higher in these stages, and so is the appearance of related damage. ATM acts in conjunction with CHK2 and p53 to block G1/S transition by inhibiting CDK2, the cycle-dependent kinase that along with Cyclin E, triggers S-phase entry [62]. CDK2 inhibition is achieved by two overlapping mechanisms that have ATM at their apex. On one hand, ATM phosphorylation of CHK2 triggers phosphorylation of CDC25A, a phosphatase required for CDK2 activation and promoting entry into S-phase [63, 64]. On the other hand, ATM-dependent activation of p53 induces upregulation of p21, which acts as a CDK2 inhibitor [65].

Replicative stresses during S-phase trigger the activation of the Intra-S-phase checkpoint to ensure that replicative stress and other types of damages do not persist in the following cell cycle stages. ATR, not ATM, is the PIKK responsible for halting the cell cycle at this stage through the activation of the intra-S-phase [61]. During this checkpoint ATR, CHK1, and p53 act together and in overlapping ways to phosphorylate CDK2, which renders it unable to form an active CDK2/cyclin A complex [63, 66]. The final result is DNA synthesis termination, premature stalling, and subsequent halt of the cell cycle.

The concerted action of ATR, CHK1, and p53 also controls the G2/M transition to ensure that no cell enters mitosis with lingering DNA damage from previous phases [67–69]. The importance of this checkpoint is highlighted by the presence of multiple overlapping and complementary mechanisms actively working together to inhibit CDK1/CyclinB1, the complex required to trigger entry into mitosis [66]. CDK1 phosphorylation has an inhibitory effect and thus, is the primary target of several of these mechanisms. After ATR-mediated activation, CHK1 phosphorylates CDC25C, a phosphatase required for CDK1 activation. Phosphorylated CDC25C binds to the 14-3-3 complex, which promotes its transport to the cytoplasm, effectively preventing CDK1 activation [70]. Active CHK1 also phosphorylates and activates WEE1, a kinase that promotes inhibitory phosphorylation of CDK1 [71]. Furthermore, ATR phosphorylates PLK1 and inhibits its role as WEE1 inhibitor, while p53 upregulates GADD45, which binds and further inhibits CDK1/CyclinB1 complex [72, 73]. Importantly, ATM also play roles in this combined effort to keep CDK1/CyclinB1 inhibited, as it can phosphorylate PLK1 and promote CHK1-mediated CDC25C phosphorylation [73, 74].

Finally, the Intra-M checkpoint is the last opportunity to prevent the transmission of damage to daughter cells. ATM and CHK1 govern this checkpoint through two distinct mechanisms that act sequentially during mitosis progression. First, inhibitory phosphorylation of PLK1 by CHK1 prevents it from acting during spindle formation and halts the cell cycle [74]. At a later point, ATR-mediated phosphorylation of Aurora B stimulates the inhibitory effect that this enzyme exerts over cytokinesis and delays exits of mitosis if the damage is detected [75].

2.3 Transcription regulation

Activation of DDR induces substantial changes to the transcriptome to equip cells with necessary tools and time to articulate a proper response. While the overall effect of DDR activation is an attenuation of global transcription and translation, many genes involved in DDR pathways must be upregulated instead [76]. For example, upregulation of XPC and other NER genes follows DDR activation, and as previously noted, DDR-mediated blocking of cell cycle progression is dependent on the induction of certain genes, namely p21 [77]. DDR exerts its influence on gene transcription through the action of several transcription factors that act as downstream effectors of DDR signaling. Some of the most important examples are p53 and BRAC1, AP-1, or E2F1. For instance, BRAC1 and p53 upregulate XPC during DDR-mediated NER upregulation; whereas, AP-1 induces the expression of XPF and XPG during the same process [76]. Other examples are p53 and AP-1 serving as transcription factors for MLH1 and MSH2—two mismatch repair genes—and E2F1 and AP-1 influencing the expression of BER components XRCC1 and APEX1, respectively.

2.4 Apoptosis and senescence

Paramount for DDR is its ability to trigger apoptosis when DNA damage is too extensive and incompatible with genome stability. Both ATM and ATR can promote apoptosis through the phosphorylation of p53, the chief regulator of apoptosis during DDR [78–80]. p53 can trigger apoptosis by playing dual roles as transcription factor activator and anti-apoptotic protein inhibitor. In the presence of unrepairable damage, p53 upregulates pro-apoptotic genes like PUMA or BAX, while binding and inhibiting anti-apoptotic proteins like BCL2 [81, 82]. In addition to apoptosis, extensive DNA damage can also induce senescence, a metabolic state that causes irreversible growth arrest [83]. Among other mechanisms, senescence can be induced during DDR by ATM and p53 upregulation of p21 [84].

2.5 Other DDR pathways

ATM and ATR also integrate into DDR several other pathways that are essential to provide an adequate and proportionate response to all kind of injuries. For instance, no proper DDR can occur without the upregulation of dNTP for DNA repair [85]. This upregulation requires tight control, as excessive dNTP production can lead to increased mutation frequency [86]. In the presence of DNA damage, DDR kinases regulate RNR—the kinase that catalyzes rate-limiting step during dNTP production—at multiple levels. For instance, p53 regulates the expression levels of RNR; whereas, ATM phosphorylation increases the stability of RNR [87]. In addition, ATR signaling inhibits degradation of some RNR subunits, further contributing to the regulation of dNTP levels by DDR kinases.

Dysfunctional telomeres can also activate ATM and ATR and elicit a response that includes halting the cell cycle and induction of senescence [88]. Telomere dysfunction can arise when errors in the Shelterin complex render telomeres unprotected. Loss of protection at telomeres can also occur by the natural attrition of telomere length experienced during DNA replication in cells that do not express telomerase [89]. In both cases, DNA ends at telomeres can be mistakenly recognized as DNA damage events and activate DDR.

Recently, activation of autophagy has emerged as another tool that DDR can use to fight severe DNA damage. While autophagy was initially thought to be exclusively activated in response to cellular damage or starvation, there is clear evidence that DNA damage can also trigger autophagy [90]. For instance, the action of mTOR—the main autophagy inhibitor—can be repressed either in an ATM or PARP1 dependent manner following DNA damage, effectively promoting autophagy [7]. Consistent with this, in response to ROS mediated damage, ATM can induce selective degradation of mitochondria by autophagy (also known as mitophagy) and pexophagy—the autophagic degradation of peroxisomes [91–93]. Integration of autophagy pathways as part of DDR repertoire may allow cells in stress to attempt pro-survival pathways first before succumbing to apoptosis.

While the complex relationships between DDR and inflammation are beginning to emerge, it is clear that ROS and other types of genomic injuries can elicit a pro-inflammatory response. As part of DDR, this pro-survival cell response is mediated mostly through ATM and PARP1 [94]. ATM directly binds and phosphorylates IKK-γ (NEMO), the regulatory subunit of the IKK complex that activates NF-kB [41]. Along with PARP1-mediated post-translational modifications, ATM phosphorylation of IKK-γ promotes activation of IKK and subsequent activation of NF-kB [41, 95–97]. Therefore, this critical pro-inflammatory enzyme is under DDR control, where it can function as a transcription factor promoting expression of pro-inflammatory cytokines and DNA repair genes [76, 94, 95, 98]. In addition, ATM is involved in a pro-inflammatory pathway known as senescence-associated secretory phenotype (SASP), a complex mechanism that secretes, among others, pro-inflammatory cytokines [94, 99].

3. Molecular basis for ataxia telangiectasia syndrome

A-T is an autosomal recessive genetic disease that affects 1 in every 40,000–100,00 births with an estimated 0.5–1% of the global population being carriers of the illness [100]. Patients confront a variety of clinical manifestations throughout their lives, with the inability to control body movements, or ataxia, being one the earliest to appear [101]. The underlying cause for the ataxia is progressive neurodegeneration, particularly of the cerebellum, which also induces dysarthria (speech difficulties), poor balance, and uncontrolled eye movements. Neurodegeneration involves the gradual disappearance of Purkinje, granular cells and the molecular layer of the cerebellar cortex, and expands to the brain stem and the spinal cord. A-T is also characterized by the presence of vascular abnormalities (telangiectasia) that manifest as red spider-like veins, present mostly in the eyes, but also found in cheeks, ears, neck, and other parts of patients' bodies [102, 103].

In addition to the ataxia and telangiectasia, A-T patients can suffer from a plethora of other clinical symptoms. They have a higher incidence of cancer, diabetes, and show premature aging. They manifest radiosensitivity, sterility, and immunodeficiencies with an elevated risk of developing autoimmune diseases such as arthritis, vitiligo, or immune thrombocytopenia [104]. Authors have also suggested that A-T patients may suffer from prolonged chronic inflammation [94]. Consistent with this, high levels of pro-inflammation cytokines are present in their serum even in the absence of infections [51, 52].

While mutations in other DDR gene can induce similar symptomatology, defective or absent, ATM is the sole genetic cause of A-T. Hundreds of pathogenic mutations have been identified in ATM from A-T patients, many of them altering splicing or causing frameshifts that result in premature termination codons. As a result, ATM is often either missing or containing truncations of different extents in A-T cells. Clinical manifestations correlate with the severity of the mutation, with milder forms of the syndrome appearing in individuals bearing mutations with mild effects on ATM function and vice versa [105].

3.1 Neurodegeneration

The most apparent clinical manifestation of the disease is probably also the most problematic to explain at the molecular level. The question of why mutations in a gene involved in DDR would have specific and discriminating effects in the neural system remains to be fully answered [5, 106]. One of the problems in answering this question is that mouse models lacking functional ATM reconstitute most of the pleiotropic effects of A-T, except for neurodegeneration [107–109].

It is clear that during neurodevelopment, rapidly dividing cells—with high energetic demands and increased mitochondria respiration—face increasing levels of threats to the integrity of their genome [110, 111]. High metabolic rates increase ROS, and produce oxidative stress, which combined with the high demand for transcription, may render these cells more susceptible to faulty DNA repair mechanisms [110, 112]. This view is consistent with the high prevalence of neurological problems in patients bearing mutations in DNA repair genes [5, 9]. Authors have proposed a model where different stages during neurodevelopment are more susceptible to mutations in different DNA repair pathways, with HR having major roles during phases of rapid proliferation—when a sister chromatid is readily available—and NHEJ being required during late development when cells undergo differentiation in G1/G0 [9]. This would explain why mutations in HR often result in embryonic lethality; whereas, mutations in some NHEJ genes present neurodevelopment problems such as microcephalia. In this model, single strand lesion repair would be required for post-developmental maintenance of neural tissue.

Cerebellum neurodegeneration in A-T patients also establishes ATM as a requirement to maintain neural tissue. The accumulation of unrepaired lesions during development—and beyond—results in degeneration problems later [113]. This is likely to happen at any tissue, but it would affect the neural system in particular, and with greater virulence, due to the longevity of its cells and the subsequent longer exposure to mutagenic agents. This injury build-up would occur progressively, mimicking the progressive nature of neurodegeneration in A-T patients.

Supporting this view, there are clear indications that neural A-T cells are under genotoxic stress. Mice cells lacking ATM gradually accumulate DSBs and show depleted levels of oxidized and reduced forms of NAD in cerebellar tissue, a hallmark of cells undergoing high levels of oxidative stress [114]. Interestingly, depletion of NAD levels only occurs in cerebellar tissues, but not in other parts of the brain, indicating that oxidative stress may be particularly acute in the cerebellum. These data are consistent with other studies that found high levels of oxidative stress in the cerebellum and Purkinje cells in particular, which likely explains the higher prevalence of neurodegeneration in the cerebellum than in other parts of the neural system [115]. The reason for the localized high levels of oxidative stress in cerebellar tissue compared to other regions of the neural system is not known, nor is the reason for the lack of a cerebellar degeneration phenotype in mice lacking ATM despite increased levels of oxidative damage.

These studies strongly suggest that the inability to repair damage caused by oxidative stress is the more plausible cause of cerebellar neurodegeneration in A-T and thus, the roles of ATM during the repair of single strand lesions may provide the molecular basis for the disease. The correlation between impaired single strand lesions repair and failure of neural tissue maintenance was further corroborated in mice that showed extensive neuron loss in the cerebellum when XRCC1 expression was selectively prevented in their brain [116]. While ATM mostly acts in DSB repair, it can also play roles during single strand lesion repair. As mentioned before, SSBs can activate ATM and promote BER by the ATM-mediated phosphorylation of XRCC1 (see Section 2.1) [46]. Whether or not, impairment of this DDR branch is related to the neurodegeneration observed in A-T remains to be elucidated.

Authors have also proposed that neurological problems arising in A-T patients may be related to the faulty resolution of R-loops in locations where active transcription is halted due to the presence of DNA lesions [9, 13]. R-loops are hybrids formed by two strands of DNA and one of RNA that are generated in a variety of circumstances and locations and are known to pose a risk to genome stability

[117]. Paused RNA polymerase sites activate ATM, which then elicit a response that includes interactions with spliceosome components that may mediate R-loop resolution [118]. In the cerebellum, the combination of high levels of oxidative stress with high demands of transcription may produce an abnormally high amount of paused transcription sites due to DNA damage. In the absence of ATM, R-loops may not be adequately resolved, eventually creating a scenario incompatible with cell life.

3.2 Telangiectasia

The localized abnormal vascular formations that A-T patients show in several parts of their bodies—particularly in the eyes—is one of the most obvious and yet least investigated phenotypes of the disease [119]. Telangiectasia is highly prevalent in A-T, only missing in patients bearing mild ATM mutations that maintain some residual protein function [120]. Very little is known about the molecular mechanism that prompts telangiectasia when ATM is absent or dysfunctional. The current model proposes that oxidative stress caused by a lack of functional ATM may upregulate HIF1A levels, a hypoxia-activated transcription factor that can induce vascularization by increasing the levels of angiogenesis factor VEGF [120]. Intriguingly, SAPS also induces secretion of VEGF, suggesting a link between this DDR controlled pathway and vascularization [121, 122].

3.3 Immunodeficiency and inflammation

A-T patients can show low levels of at least one type of immunoglobulin, inadequate antibody responses to infections and abnormal T and B lymphocyte counts [123, 124]. These phenotypes can be attributed to the roles that ATM has in regulating NHEJ during V(D)J recombination and class-switch recombination (CSR), two recombination processes required to produce antibody diversity during adaptive immunity. Both V(D)J and CSR involve induction of programmed DSBs followed by ATM-aided NHEJ repair [125]. For instance, during V(D)J ATM localizes to break sites and regulate NHEJ components, while p53BP1 phosphorylation by ATM is a crucial event during CSR. The regulatory roles that ATM exerts on these two processes are likely to be extensive and involve other DDR pathways. In A-T patients with immunodeficiencies, programmed DSBs remain unrepaired, and their persistence can cause severe T and B-cell developmental problems [126–128].

There is growing evidence that the innate immune response may be tightly linked to several clinical manifestations observed in A-T patients. Lack of ATM creates high levels of ROS and oxidative damage, which is known to induce pro-inflammatory cytokines [111, 129, 130]. ATM-deficient cells cannot trigger pexophagy and other forms of autophagy to counteract the negatives effect of oxidative damage, further compounding the problem [91]. Persistent genotoxic stress can, therefore, create chronic inflammation in A-T patients, a condition linked to several A-T symptoms: increased levels of cardiovascular and autoimmune diseases, insulin resistance, and aging. Tellingly, the immune response contributes to neurodegeneration during Alzheimer's disease, possibly suggesting that in A-T patients, chronic inflammation may also contribute to neurodegeneration in cerebellar tissues suffering high levels of genotoxic stress [131].

3.4 Radiosensitivity and increased cancer risk

Several DDR pathways contribute to the increased cancer risk seen in A-T patients. The inability of A-T cells to coordinate DNA repair with other DDR pathways can leave unrepaired genomic injuries and elevate the number of mutations in cells—including perilous DSBs—rendering cells highly sensitive to ionizing radiation. Lack of ATM permits these mutations to escape cell cycle checkpoints control and be transmitted to daughter cells, further contributing to tumorigenesis. This process can continue unchecked, as the genomic instability that it produces does not trigger apoptosis when ATM is absent or dysfunctional.

One of the most common malignancies in A-T patients is breast cancer [132]. Even heterozygous individuals bearing debilitating mutations in just one of the ATM genes also have increased breast cancer incidence. While many DDR components are likely to participate in breast cancer tumorigenesis, the loss of the direct control that ATM exerts over BRAC1 is likely one of the major contributing factors. Lymphomas of B-cell origin and leukemia of T-cell origin are also very common in A-T patients, as unrepaired programmed DSBs persisting in developing T and B cells can often be the substrate of translocations [133].

3.5 Other clinical features

Both male and female A-T patients show infertility due to abnormal meiosis progression. During meiosis, ATM controls the number of DSBs created by SPO11 and ensures their even distribution in the genome [134]. This is achieved by recruiting ATM to SPO11-generated DSBs, which inhibits the formation of further cuts in the vicinity of break sites. Mice models have shown a meiotic arrest in prophase I, faulty synapsis, and chromosome fragmentation leading to massive germ cell loss [107, 135], suggesting that the loss of ATM's roles during meiosis is the underlying cause of infertility in A-T patients.

A-T patients can suffer from insulin resistance and thus, have a higher risk of developing diabetes, a clinical feature that they share with carriers of the disease. The cause for this phenotype is likely to be multifactorial, but it is well-defined that ATM phosphorylates several targets—e.g., translation regulation 4E-BP1—in response to insulin [25]. Furthermore, a lack of fully functional ATM correlates with an inhibition of IRS1 (insulin receptor substrate 1) and low levels of IGF1-R (insulin-like growth factor1 receptor), suggesting possible mechanisms causing this clinical feature [94, 136, 137].

4. Conclusion

While much progress has been made to understand A-T at the molecular level, there are still important questions that remain unanswered. This is especially true for the cerebellar neurodegeneration observed in A-T patients, where unknown tissue-specific factors may be at play. The genesis and the extent of some of the A-T clinical features are likely to be the result of interwoven relationships between many pathways and pathologies described in here and hence, elucidating their connections will be crucial to fully understand the disease and develop effective tools for its treatment.

Acknowledgements

This manuscript was funded and supported by the Smith Chair in Biology at the University of St. Thomas.

Conflict of interest

I have no conflict of interest to declare.

Author details

Albert Ribes-Zamora
Biology Department, University of St. Thomas, Houston, USA

*Address all correspondence to: ribesza@stthom.edu

References

[1] Jackson SP, Bartek J. The DNA-damage response in human biology and disease. Nature. 2009

[2] Sancar A, Lindsey-Boltz LA, Ünsal-Kaçmaz K, Linn S. Molecular mechanisms of mammalian DNA repair and the DNA damage checkpoints. Annual Review of Biochemistry. 2004

[3] Sirbu BM, Cortez D. DNA damage response: Three levels of DNA repair regulation. Cold Spring Harbor Perspectives in Biology. 2013

[4] Ciccia A, Elledge SJ. The DNA damage response: Making it safe to play with knives. Molecular Cell. 2010

[5] Coon EA, Benarroch EE. DNA damage response selected review and neurologic implications. Neurology. 2018

[6] Harper JW, Elledge SJ. The DNA damage response: Ten years after. Molecular Cell. 2007

[7] Cartwright BM, Musich PR, Zou Y. DNA damage: Cellular responses, repair and cancer treatment. In: Regulation of Signal Transduction in Human Cell. Singapore: Springer Nature; 2018. pp. 99-127

[8] Shibata A, Jeggo PA. DNA double-strand break repair in a cellular context. Clinical Oncology. 2014

[9] Rulten SL, Caldecott KW. DNA strand break repair and neurodegeneration. DNA Repair (Amst). 2013

[10] Enriquez-Rios V, Dumitrache LC, Downing SM, Li Y, Brown EJ, Russell HR, et al. DNA-PKcs, ATM, and ATR interplay maintains genome integrity during neurogenesis. The Journal of Neuroscience. 2017

[11] Stracker TH, Roig I, Knobel PA, Marjanović M. The ATM signaling network in development and disease. Frontiers in Genetics. 2013

[12] Kulkarni A, Wilson DM. The involvement of DNA-damage and -repair defects in neurological dysfunction. American Journal of Human Genetics. 2008

[13] Blackford AN, Jackson SP. ATM, ATR, and DNA-PK: The trinity at the heart of the DNA damage response. Molecular Cell. 2017

[14] Rass U, Ahel I, West SC. Defective DNA repair and neurodegenerative disease. Cell. 2007

[15] Antoccia A, Kobayashi J, Tauchi H, Matsuura S, Komatsu K. Nijmegen breakage syndrome and functions of the responsible protein, NBS1. Genome Dynamics. 2006

[16] O'Driscoll M, Ruiz-Perez VL, Woods CG, Jeggo PA, Goodship JA. A splicing mutation affecting expression of ataxia-telangiectasia and Rad3-related protein [ATR] results in Seckel syndrome. Nature Genetics. 2003

[17] Zhou Y, Lee JH, Jiang W, Crowe JL, Zha S, Paull TT. Regulation of the DNA damage response by DNA-PKcs inhibitory phosphorylation of ATM. Molecular Cell. 2017

[18] Kozlov SV, Graham ME, Jakob B, Tobias F, Kijas AW, Tanuji M, et al. Autophosphorylation and ATM activation: Additional sites add to the complexity. The Journal of Biological Chemistry. 2011

[19] Bakkenist CJ, Kastan MB. DNA damage activates ATM through intermolecular autophosphorylation and dimer dissociation. Nature. 2003

[20] Lavin MF, Kozlov S. ATM activation and DNA damage response. Cell Cycle. 2007

[21] Bannister AJ, Gottlieb TM, Kouzarides T, Jackson SP. c-Jun is phosphorylated by the DNA-dependent protein kinase in vitro; definition of the minimal kinase recognition motif. Nucleic Acids Research. 1993

[22] Traven A, Heierhorst J. SQ/TQ cluster domains: Concentrated ATM/ATR kinase phosphorylation site regions in DNA-damage-response proteins. BioEssays. 2005

[23] Cheung HC, San Lucas FA, Hicks S, Chang K, Bertuch AA, Ribes-Zamora A. An S/T-Q cluster domain census unveils new putative targets under Tel1/Mec1 control. BMC Genomics. 2012

[24] Cara L, Baitemirova M, Follis J, Larios-Sanz M, Ribes-Zamora A. The ATM- and ATR-related SCD domain is over-represented in proteins involved in nervous system development. Scientific Reports. 2016

[25] Matsuoka S, Ballif BA, Smogorzewska A, McDonald ER, Hurov KE, Luo J, et al. ATM and ATR substrate analysis reveals extensive protein networks responsive to DNA damage. Science. 2007

[26] Matsuoka S, Rotman G, Ogawa A, Shiloh Y, Tamai K, Elledge SJ. Ataxia telangiectasia-mutated phosphorylates Chk2 in vivo and in vitro. Proceedings of the National Academy of Sciences. 2000

[27] Matsuoka S, Huang M, Elledge SJ. Linkage of ATM to cell cycle regulation by the Chk2 protein kinase. Science. 1998

[28] Banin S, Moyal L, Shieh SY, Taya Y, Anderson CW, Chessa L, et al. Enhanced phosphorylation of p53 by ATM in response to DNA damage. Science. 1998

[29] Guo Z, Kozlov S, Lavin MF, Person MD, Paull TT. ATM activation by oxidative stress. Science. 2010

[30] Ray Chaudhuri A, Nussenzweig A. The multifaceted roles of PARP1 in DNA repair and chromatin remodelling. Nature Reviews. Molecular Cell Biology. 2017

[31] Wei H, Yu X. Functions of PARylation in DNA damage repair pathways. Genomics, Proteomics & Bioinformatics. 2016

[32] Williams GJ, Lees-Miller SP, Tainer JA. Mre11-Rad50-Nbs1 conformations and the control of sensing, signaling, and effector responses at DNA double-strand breaks. DNA Repair. 2010

[33] Wang H, Shi LZ, Wong CCL, Han X, Hwang PYH, Truong LN, et al. The interaction of CtIP and Nbs1 connects CDK and ATM to regulate HR-mediated double-strand break repair. PLoS Genetics. 2013

[34] Rogakou EP, Pilch DR, Orr AH, Ivanova VS, Bonner WM. DNA double-stranded breaks induce histone H2AX phosphorylation on serine 139. The Journal of Biological Chemistry. 1998

[35] Stucki M, Clapperton JA, Mohammad D, Yaffe MB, Smerdon SJ, Jackson SP. MDC1 directly binds phosphorylated histone H2AX to regulate cellular responses to DNA double-strand breaks. Cell. 2005

[36] Jungmichel S, Clapperton JA, Lloyd J, Hari FJ, Spycher C, Pavic L, et al. The molecular basis of ATM-dependent dimerization of the Mdc1 DNA damage checkpoint mediator. Nucleic Acids Research. 2012

[37] Adams KE, Medhurst AL, Dart DA, Lakin ND. Recruitment of ATR to sites of ionising radiation-induced DNA damage requires ATM and components of the MRN protein complex. Oncogene. 2006

[38] Shibata A, Conrad S, Birraux J, Geuting V, Barton O, Ismail A, et al. Factors determining DNA double-strand break repair pathway choice in G2 phase. The EMBO Journal. 2011

[39] Chapman JR, Taylor MRG, Boulton SJ. Playing the end game: DNA double-Strand break repair pathway choice. Molecular Cell. 2012

[40] Xu B, O'Donnell AH, Kim ST, Kastan MB. Phosphorylation of serine 1387 in Brca1 is specifically required for the ATM-mediated S-phase checkpoint after ionizing irradiation. Cancer Research. 2002

[41] Wu ZH, Shi Y, Tibbetts RS, Miyamoto S. Molecular linkage between the kinase ATM and NF-κB signaling in response to genotoxic stimuli. Science. 2006

[42] Sartori AA, Lukas C, Coates J, Mistrik M, Fu S, Bartek J, et al. Human CtIP promotes DNA end resection. Nature. 2007

[43] Jowsey PA, Doherty AJ, Rouse J. Human PTIP facilitates ATM-mediated activation of p53 and promotes cellular resistance to ionizing radiation. The Journal of Biological Chemistry. 2004

[44] Hustedt N, Durocher D. The control of DNA repair by the cell cycle. Nature Cell Biology. 2017

[45] Jiang W, Crowe JL, Liu X, Nakajima S, Wang Y, Li C, et al. Differential phosphorylation of DNA-PKcs regulates the interplay between end-processing and end-ligation during nonhomologous end-joining. Molecular Cell. 2015

[46] Chou WC, Hu LY, Hsiung CN, Shen CY. Initiation of the ATM-Chk2 DNA damage response through the base excision repair pathway. Carcinogenesis. 2015

[47] Wilson DM, Bohr VA. The mechanics of base excision repair, and its relationship to aging and disease. DNA Repair (Amst). 2007

[48] Wu X, Shell SM, Yang Z, Zou Y. Phosphorylation of nucleotide excision repair factor xeroderma pigmentosum group A by ataxia telangiectasia mutated and Rad3-related-dependent checkpoint pathway promotes cell survival in response to UV irradiation. Cancer Research. 2006

[49] Shell SM, Li Z, Shkriabai N, Kvaratskhelia M, Brossey C, Serrano MA, et al. Checkpoint kinase ATR promotes nucleotide excision repair of UV-induced DNA damage via physical interaction withxeroderma pigmentosum group a. The Journal of Biological Chemistry. 2009

[50] Barckhausen C, Roos WP, Naumann SC, Kaina B. Malignant melanoma cells acquire resistance to DNA interstrand cross-linking chemotherapeutics by p53-triggered upregulation of DDB2/XPC-mediated DNA repair. Oncogene. 2014

[51] Wang XW, Yeh H, Schaeffer L, Roy R, Moncollin V, Egly JM, et al. p53 modulation of TFIIH-associated nucleotide excision repair activity. Nature Genetics. 1995

[52] Wang QE, Zhu Q, Wani MA, Wani G, Chen J, Wani AA. Tumor suppressor p53 dependent recruitment of nucleotide excision repair factors XPC and TFIIH to DNA damage. DNA Repair (Amst). 2003

[53] Singh TR, Ali AM, Paramasivam M, Pradhan A, Wahengbam K, Seidman MM, et al. ATR-dependent phosphorylation of FANCM at serine 1045 is essential for FANCM functions. Cancer Research. 2013

[54] Collins NB, Wilson JB, Bush T, Thomashevski A, Roberts KJ, Jones NJ,

et al. ATR-dependent phosphorylation of FANCA on serine 1449 after DNA damage is important for FA pathway function. Blood. 2009

[55] Ceccaldi R, Sarangi P, D'Andrea AD. The Fanconi anaemia pathway: New players and new functions. Nature Reviews. Molecular Cell Biology. 2016

[56] Offer H, Zurer I, Banfalvi G, Reha'K M, Falcovitz A, Milyavsky M, et al. p53 modulates base excision repair activity in a cell cycle-specific manner after genotoxic stress. Cancer Research. 2001

[57] Zurer I, Hofseth LJ, Cohen Y, Xu-Welliver M, Hussain SP, Harris CC, et al. The role of p53 in base excision repair following genotoxic stress. Carcinogenesis. 2004

[58] Romanova LY, Willers H, Blagosklonny MV, Powell SN. The interaction of p53 with replication protein a mediates suppression of homologous recombination. Oncogene. 2004

[59] Ammazzalorso F, Pirzio LM, Bignami M, Franchitto A, Pichierri P. ATR and ATM differently regulate WRN to prevent DSBs at stalled replication forks and promote replication fork recovery. The EMBO Journal. 2010

[60] Croteau DL, Popuri V, Opresko PL, Bohr VA. Human RecQ helicases in DNA repair, recombination, and replication. Annual Review of Biochemistry. 2014

[61] Liu M, Hu WX. Cell cycle checkpoint signaling through the ATR and ATM kinases. In: 2nd International Conference on Information Science and Engineering, ICISE2010 – Proceedings; 2010

[62] Bartek J, Lukas J. Mammalian G1- and S-phase checkpoints in response to DNA damage. Current Opinion in Cell Biology. 2001

[63] Xiao Z, Chen Z, Gunasekera AH, Sowin TJ, Rosenberg SH, Fesik S, et al. Chk1 mediates S and G2 arrests through Cdc25A degradation in response to DNA-damaging agents. The Journal of Biological Chemistry. 2003

[64] Mailand N, Falck J, Lukas C, Syljuåsen RG, Welcker M, Bartek J, et al. Rapid destruction of human Cdc25A in response to DNA damage. Science. 2000

[65] Abbas T, Dutta A. P21 in cancer: Intricate networks and multiple activities. Nature Reviews. Cancer. 2009

[66] Bartek J, Lukas J. Chk1 and Chk2 kinases in checkpoint control and cancer. Cancer Cell. 2003

[67] Liu S, Shiotani B, Lahiri M, Maréchal A, Tse A, Leung CCY, et al. ATR autophosphorylation as a molecular switch for checkpoint activation. Molecular Cell. 2011

[68] Sanchez Y, Bachant J, Wang H, Hu F, Liu D, Tetzlaff M, et al. Control of the DNA damage checkpoint by Chk1 and Rad53 protein kinases through distinct mechanisms. Science. 1999

[69] Sanchez Y, Wong C, Thoma RS, Richman R, Wu Z, Piwnica-Worms H, et al. Conservation of the Chk1 checkpoint pathway in mammals: Linkage of DNA damage to Cdk regulation through Cdc25. Science. 1997

[70] Peng CY, Graves PR, Thoma RS, Wu Z, Shaw AS, Piwnica-Worms H. Mitotic and G2 checkpoint control: Regulation of 14-3-3 protein binding by phosphorylation of Cdc25c on serine-216. Science. 1997

[71] Lee J, Kumagai A, Dunphy WG. Positive regulation of Wee1 by Chk1 and 14-3-3 proteins. Molecular Biology of the Cell. 2001

[72] Yang Q, Manicone A, Coursen JD, Linke SP, Nagashima M, Forgues M,

et al. Identification of a functional domain in a GADD45-mediated G2/M checkpoint. The Journal of Biological Chemistry. 2000

[73] Harvey SL, Charlet A, Haas W, Gygi SP, Kellogg DR. Cdk1-dependent regulation of the mitotic inhibitor Wee1. Cell. 2005

[74] Zitouni S, Nabais C, Jana SC, Guerrero A, Bettencourt-Dias M. Polo-like kinases: Structural variations lead to multiple functions. Nature Reviews. Molecular Cell Biology. 2014

[75] Mackay DR, Ullman KS. ATR and a Chk1-Aurora B pathway coordinate postmitotic genome surveillance with cytokinetic abscission. Molecular Biology of the Cell. 2015

[76] Christmann M, Kaina B. Transcriptional regulation of human DNA repair genes following genotoxic stress: Trigger mechanisms, inducible responses and genotoxic adaptation. Nucleic Acids Research. 2013

[77] Adimoolam S, Ford JM. p53 and DNA damage-inducible expression of the xeroderma pigmentosum group C gene. Proceedings of the National Academy of Sciences. 2002

[78] Jenkins LMM, Durell SR, Mazur SJ, Appella E. p53 N-terminal phosphorylation: A defining layer of complex regulation. Carcinogenesis. 2012

[79] Gannon HS, Woda BA, Jones SN. ATM phosphorylation of Mdm2 Ser394 regulates the amplitude and duration of the DNA damage response in mice. Cancer Cell. 2012

[80] Vousden KH, Lane DP. p53 in health and disease. Nature Reviews. Molecular Cell Biology. 2007

[81] Nakano K, Vousden KH. PUMA, a novel proapoptotic gene, is induced by p53. Molecular Cell. 2001

[82] Wu Y, Mehew JW, Heckman CA, Arcinas M, Boxer LM. Negative regulation of bcl-2 expression by p53 in hematopoietic cells. Oncogene. 2001

[83] Shimizu I, Yoshida Y, Suda M, Minamino T. DNA damage response and metabolic disease. Cell Metabolism. 2014

[84] Jackson JG, Pereira-Smith OM. p53 is preferentially recruited to the promoters of growth arrest genes p21 and GADD45 during replicative senescence of normal human fibroblasts. Cancer Research. 2006

[85] Elledge SJ, Zhou Z, Allen JB, Navas TA. DNA damage and cell cycle regulation of ribonucleotide reductase. BioEssays. 1993

[86] Chabes A, Georgieva B, Domkin V, Zhao X, Rothstein R, Thelander L. Survival of DNA damage in yeast directly depends on increased dNTP levels allowed by relaxed feedback inhibition of ribonucleotide reductase. Cell. 2003

[87] Tanaka H, Arakawa H, Yamaguchi T, Shiraishi K, Fukuda S, Matsui K, et al. A ribonucleotide reductase gene involved in a p53-dependent cell-cycle checkpoint for DNA damage. Nature. 2000

[88] de Lange T. Shelterin-mediated telomere protection. Annual Review of Genetics. 2018

[89] Reaper PM, Clay-Farrace L, Fiegler H, Carr P, Von Zglinicki T, Saretzki G, et al. A DNA damage checkpoint response in telomere-initiated senescence. Nature. 2003

[90] Abedin MJ, Wang D, McDonnell MA, Lehmann U, Kelekar A. Autophagy delays apoptotic death in breast cancer cells following DNA damage. Cell Death and Differentiation. 2007

[91] Zhang J, Tripathi DN, Jing J, Alexander A, Kim J, Powell RT, et al.

ATM functions at the peroxisome to induce pexophagy in response to ROS. Nature Cell Biology. 2015

[92] Valentin-Vega YA, Kastan MB. A new role for ATM: Regulating mitochondrial function and mitophagy. Autophagy. 2012

[93] Valentin-Vega YA, MacLean KH, Tait-Mulder J, Milasta S, Steeves M, Dorsey FC, et al. Mitochondrial dysfunction in ataxia-telangiectasia. Blood. 2012

[94] Zaki-Dizaji M, Akrami SM, Azizi G, Abolhassani H, Aghamohammadi A. Inflammation, a significant player of ataxia–telangiectasia pathogenesis? Inflammation Research. 2018

[95] Hellweg CE. The nuclear factor κB pathway: A link to the immune system in the radiation response. Cancer Letters. 2015

[96] Hadian K, Krappmann D, Hayden MS, Ghosh S, Vallabhapurapu S, Karin M, et al. Signals from the nucleus: Activation of NF-kappaB by cytosolic ATM in the DNA damage response. Science Signaling. 2011

[97] Stilmann M, Hinz M, Arslan SÇ, Zimmer A, Schreiber V, Scheidereit C. A nuclear poly[ADP-ribose]-dependent signalosome confers DNA damage-induced IκB kinase activation. Molecular Cell. 2009

[98] Miyamoto S. Nuclear initiated NF-κB signaling: NEMO and ATM take center stage. Cell Research. 2011

[99] Kang C, Xu Q, Martin TD, Li MZ, Demaria M, Aron L, et al. The DNA damage response induces inflammation and senescence by inhibiting autophagy of GATA4. Science. 2015

[100] Zaki-Dizaji M, Akrami SM, Abolhassani H, Rezaei N, Aghamohammadi A. Ataxia telangiectasia syndrome: Moonlighting ATM. Expert Review of Clinical Immunology. 2017

[101] Chun HH, Gatti RA. Ataxia-telangiectasia, an evolving phenotype. DNA Repair. 2004

[102] Verhagen MMM, Abdo WF, Willemsen MAAP, Hogervorst FBL, Smeets DFCM, Hiel JAP, et al. Clinical spectrum of ataxia-telangiectasia in adulthood. Neurology. 2009

[103] Taylor AMR, Harnden DG, Arlett CF, Harcourt SA, Lehmann AR, Stevens S, et al. Ataxia telangiectasia: A human mutation with abnormal radiation sensitivity. Nature. 1975

[104] Ammann AJ, Hong R. Autoimmune phenomena in ataxia telangiectasia. The Journal of Pediatrics. 1971

[105] Verhagen MMM, Last JI, Hogervorst FBL, Smeets DFCM, Roeleveld N, Verheijen F, et al. Presence of ATM protein and residual kinase activity correlates with the phenotype in ataxia-telangiectasia: A genotype-phenotype study. Human Mutation. 2012

[106] Biton S, Barzilai A, Shiloh Y. The neurological phenotype of ataxia-telangiectasia: Solving a persistent puzzle. DNA Repair (Amst). 2008

[107] Barlow C, Hirotsune S, Paylor R, Liyanage M, Eckhaus M, Collins F, et al. Atm-deficient mice: A paradigm of ataxia telangiectasia. Cell. 1996

[108] Elson A, Wang Y, Daugherty CJ, Morton CC, Zhou F, Campos-Torres J, et al. Pleiotropic defects in ataxia-telangiectasia protein-deficient mice. Proceedings of the National Academy of Sciences. 1996

[109] Xu Y, Ashley T, Brainerd EE, Bronson RT, Meyn MS, Baltimore D. Targeted disruption of ATM leads to growth retardation, chromosomal

fragmentation during meiosis, immune defects, and thymic lymphoma. Genes & Development. 1996

[110] Barlow C, Dennery PA, Shigenaga MK, Smith MA, Morrow JD, Roberts LJ, et al. Loss of the ataxia–telangiectasia gene product causes oxidative damage in target organs. Neurobiology. 1999

[111] Kamsler A, Daily D, Hochman A, Stern N, Shiloh Y, Rotman G, et al. Increased oxidative stress in ataxia telangiectasia evidenced by alterations in redox state of brains from ATM-deficient mice. Cancer Research. 2001

[112] Weissman L, de Souza-Pinto NC, Stevnsner T, Bohr VA. DNA repair, mitochondria, and neurodegeneration. Neuroscience. 2007

[113] Rutten BPF, Schmitz C, Gerlach OHH, Oyen HM, de Mesquita EB, Steinbusch HWM, et al. The aging brain: Accumulation of dna damage or neuron loss? Neurobiology of Aging. 2007

[114] Stern N, Hochman A, Zemach N, Weizman N, Hammel I, Shiloh Y, et al. Accumulation of DNA damage and reduced levels of nicotine adenine dinucleotide in the brains of ATM-deficient mice. The Journal of Biological Chemistry. 2002

[115] Yang Y, Hui CW, Li J, Herrup K. The interaction of the ATM genotype with inflammation and oxidative stress. PLoS One. 2014

[116] Lee Y, Katyal S, Li Y, El-Khamisy SF, Russell HR, Caldecott KW, et al. The genesis of cerebellar interneurons and the prevention of neural DNA damage require XRCC1. Nature Neuroscience. 2009

[117] Aguilera A, García-Muse T. R loops: From transcription byproducts to threats to genome stability. Molecular Cell. 2012

[118] Tresini M, Warmerdam DO, Kolovos P, Snijder L, Vrouwe MG, Demmers JAA, et al. The core spliceosome as target and effector of non-canonical ATM signalling. Nature. 2015

[119] Kamiya M, Yamanouchi H, Yoshida T, Arai H, Yokoo H, Sasaki A, et al. Ataxia telangiectasia with vascular abnormalities in the brain parenchyma: Report of an autopsy case and literature review. Pathology International. 2001

[120] Schoenaker MHD, Van Os NJH, Van der Flier M, Van Deuren M, Seyger MM, Taylor AMR, et al. Telangiectasias in ataxia telangiectasia: Clinical significance, role of ATM deficiency and potential pathophysiological mechanisms. European Journal of Medical Genetics. 2018

[121] Kuilman T, Michaloglou C, Vredeveld LCW, Douma S, van Doorn R, Desmet CJ, et al. Oncogene-induced senescence relayed by an interleukin-dependent inflammatory network. Cell. 2008

[122] Acosta JC, O'Loghlen A, Banito A, Guijarro MV, Augert A, Raguz S, et al. Chemokine signaling via the CXCR2 receptor reinforces senescence. Cell. 2008

[123] Driessen GJ, Ijspeert H, Weemaes CMR, Haraldsson Á, Trip M, Warris A, et al. Antibody deficiency in patients with ataxia telangiectasia is caused by disturbed B- and T-cell homeostasis and reduced immune repertoire diversity. The Journal of Allergy and Clinical Immunology. 2013

[124] Nowak-Wegrzyn A, Crawford TO, Winkelstein JA, Carson KA, Lederman HM. Immunodeficiency and infections in ataxia-telangiectasia. Journal of Pediatrics. 2004

[125] Bassing CH, Swat W, Alt FW. The mechanism and regulation of

chromosomal V[D]J recombination. Cell. 2002

[126] Ghiasy S, Parvaneh L, Azizi G, Sadri G, Zaki dizaji M, Abolhassani H, et al. The clinical significance of complete class switching defect in Ataxia telangiectasia patients. Expert Review of Clinical Immunology. 2017

[127] Kraus M, Lev A, Simon AJ, Levran I, Nissenkorn A, Levi YB, et al. Disturbed B and T cell homeostasis and neogenesis in patients with ataxia telangiectasia. Journal of Clinical Immunology. 2014

[128] Bredemeyer AL, Huang C-Y, Walker LM, Bassing CH, Sleckman BP. Aberrant V[D]J recombination in ataxia telangiectasia mutated-deficient lymphocytes is dependent on nonhomologous DNA end joining. Journal of Immunology. 2008

[129] Rodier F, Coppé JP, Patil CK, Hoeijmakers WAM, Muñoz DP, Raza SR, et al. Persistent DNA damage signalling triggers senescence-associated inflammatory cytokine secretion. Nature Cell Biology. 2009

[130] Rodier F, Munoz DP, Teachenor R, Chu V, Le O, Bhaumik D, et al. DNA-SCARS: Distinct nuclear structures that sustain damage-induced senescence growth arrest and inflammatory cytokine secretion. Journal of Cell Science. 2011

[131] Fakhoury M. Role of immunity and inflammation in the pathophysiology of neurodegenerative diseases. Neurodegenerative Diseases. 2015

[132] Estiar MA, Mehdipour P. ATM in breast and brain tumors: A comprehensive review. Cancer Biology & Medicine. 2018

[133] Nussenzweig A, Nussenzweig MC. Origin of chromosomal translocations in lymphoid cancer. Cell. 2010

[134] Lange J, Pan J, Cole F, Thelen MP, Jasin M, Keeney S. ATM controls meiotic double-strand-break formation. Nature. 2011

[135] Hamer G, Kal HB, Westphal CH, Ashley T, de Rooij DG. Ataxia telangiectasia mutated expression and activation in the Testis1. Biology of Reproduction. 2004

[136] Macaulay VM, Salisbury AJ, Bohula EA, Playford MP, Smorodinsky NI, Shiloh Y. Downregulation of the type 1 insulin-like growth factor receptor in mouse melanoma cells is associated with enhanced radiosensitivity and impaired activation of ATM kinase. Oncogene. 2001

[137] Ching JK, Luebbert SH, Collins RL IV, Zhang Z, Marupudi N, Banerjee S, et al. Ataxia telangiectasia mutated impacts insulin-like growth factor 1 signalling in skeletal muscle. Experimental Physiology. 2013

Section 4

Reading and Neurodevelopmental Disorder

Chapter 6

The Neurobiological Development of Reading Fluency

Bobbie Jean Koen

Abstract

This chapter offers an extensive review of current and foundational research literature on the neurodevelopment of dyslexia and reading fluency worldwide. The impact of different languages and their orthographies on the acquisition of phonological analysis and orthographical features by beginning readers is explored. Contributions from the Psycholinguistic Grain Size Theory and new assessments, i.e. rapid automatized naming, have focused and advanced the understanding of slow phonological and visual processing skills. Recently, the development of new definitions of fluency has led to a proposed continuum of automatized decoding and processing skills required for students of English. Computer technology has enhanced the use of visual hemisphere-specific stimulation to affect the neurodevelopment of efficient word retrieval pathways and to increase reading speed. Processes for subtyping students based on reading behaviors and then stimulating a particular hemisphere of the brain with the fast presentation of words and phrases have been found to change levels of activation in key brain locations and increase the fluent processing of connected text. Newer technologies such as diffusion tensor imaging, while somewhat suspect, may provide the evidence that ultimately will document the changes in communication between regions of interest regulating the automaticity of brain functions in reading.

Keywords: dyslexia, rapid automatized naming (RAN), phonological processing, visual processing, visual hemisphere-specific stimulation (VHSS), fluency

1. Introduction

The worldwide narrative around fluency has grown dramatically in the last 10 years. This surge in interest has been driven, perhaps, by new working definitions of fluency, and the growing realization that different languages pose variable challenges to students with dyslexia who exhibit problems with reading fluency. While analyzing their own language's nuances, researchers have inundated these students with behavioral measures of nonverbal and verbal intelligence, reading accuracy, phonological skill, spelling, orthographic patterns, short-term memory, vocabulary – receptive and expressive, visual information processing and memory, and speed of processing. Through these various behavioral assessments, the strengths and weaknesses of struggling readers of every language are quantified, modeled and correlated to describe the multitude of possible different literacy actions displayed.

It seems inevitable that some kind of labels would need to be created to identify these special readers. The dual route model of reading constitutes the background of dyslexia subtyping [1]. Its central axiom is that no single processing procedure produces the correct pronunciations of both nonwords or pseudo-words (e.g. slint) and exception or irregular words (e.g. pint) [2]. It is theorized that nonwords can only be correctly pronounced using the grapheme-phoneme correspondence rules, the "non-lexical" route; exception words require an additional procedure, the "lexical" route, because they cannot be pronounced by the rules and readers must use context to figure them out. In many studies, subjects are classified in terms of accuracy either as "phonological dyslexics" when pseudo-word reading ability is impaired but irregular word reading is spared, or as "surface dyslexics" when the reverse occurs- irregular word reading is compromised while pseudo-word reading is intact [3]. For example, in accuracy-based studies in Spanish, surface dyslexics were more frequent than phonological dyslexics [4]. However unlike English, most orthographies have highly regular grapheme-phoneme correspondences with relatively few "exception" words [5], so the applicability of the dual-route framework beyond English has been questioned [6]. More recently, researchers have focused on those children who display Single Deficits (phonological processing weakness) and those who have the dreaded Double Deficit or Double Dissociation (phonological processing and processing speed deficits) [7]. They have worked hard comparing disabled reading and cognitive skill performances with normal readers who are carefully matched by chronological age or reading level (reading age), who are younger, or who represent a different ethnicity. The subtyping, use of labels, and multi-control-group comparisons all serve to refine and focus the discussion of how these students learn to read fluently or not.

To a lesser extent, investigators have used neurobiological technology to explore various brain activations: post-mortem studies of brains of individuals with dyslexia [8], Magnetoencephalography (MEG) and Magnetic Source Imaging (MSI) to provide information both on the spatial localization and on the timing of neurophysiological processes [9], positron emission topography (PET) to examine differences in resting state blood flow in regions of interest in the brain [10], and computerized tomography (CT) and structural magnetic resonance imaging (MRI) to examine noninvasively structural brain differences [11]. Decreased activation in the left temporal–parietal cortex of adults with dyslexia was first found using functional magnetic resonance imaging (fMRI) by Constable et al. [12]. These technologies were developed and implemented in an effort to understand better the growth of the phonological and visual processing systems and verbal retrieval systems in beginning learners that for many readers seem automatic. The crucial issue is the reliability of the different sub-types, which differ according to the type of response taken into account (accuracy, speed, or both) and the type of orthography (opaque/transparent) being evaluated [13].

2. Considerations for expressions of dyslexia

It is clear that depending on what is emphasized in any given language (e.g. fluency in German; visual–spatial memory in Chinese; phonological skills in English), there will be somewhat different manifestations of dyslexia, as well as different predictors of reading failure. Cross-language studies highlight the importance, not only of regular language features, but also the influence of the writing system (orthography) on reading performance [14]. The type of orthography that the child is acquiring is a primary cultural factor that influences reading acquisition in both typical and atypical development [15]. It has been considered that the cognitive processes underpinning reading ability may be differently involved in producing the symptoms of Developmental Dyslexia, depending on orthographic transparency [16]. Generally, languages that are considered more transparent with regular orthographies are Spanish, German, Finnish, Dutch, Greek, Italian and Hebrew, while English and French are considered less regular and therefore, more opaque.

A particularly challenging example is found in the standard Arabic language. Most Arabic words are morphologically derived from roots and written Arabic uses three basic diacritical marks corresponding to short vowels. Arabic script is also made with different degrees of internal connectivity or ligation between the letters within a word. In Algeria, standard Arabic is the first written language taught in the first 3 years of schooling, and there is a transition from vowelized to un-vowelized forms of reading starting from the third grade. Although the vowelized form of Arabic is highly transparent, the non-vowelized form is rather opaque [13]. Clearly, even though the language itself is fairly regular, the features of orthography present unique difficulties to students.

A central hypothesis in the area of reading accuracy and speed across orthographies is the Psycholinguistic Grain Size Theory of reading. This idea suggests that differences in reading accuracy and speed across orthographies reflect basic differences in the nature of the phonological recoding and reading strategies [17]. Learning to read in orthographically inconsistent languages cannot rely on letter to sound correspondences (small grain size), forcing the reader to develop flexible unit size recoding strategies, such as morphological units, analogy and whole-word recognition. It would follow that these processing differences would also reflect variable activations in key processing areas in the brain. This theory would seem to impact the less regular features of a language and, particularly, languages such as English and French that are highly irregular and opaque.

Another important idea in this field is the growing body of work demonstrating the predictive ability of "rapid automatized naming" or RAN tasks [18] in reading performance. Several researchers have used these tasks where children are presented with separate arrays of different primary colors, common objects, numerals from 0 to 9, and/or single letters, and are timed while they name the stimuli as quickly as they can. It has been claimed that RAN, and in particular, the RAN alphanumeric component (digit naming and letter naming), is associated with reading success [19]. A predominate and somewhat controversial view is that reading and RAN could be linked together through the general phonological processing system because they both tap the speed of accessing phonological representations in long-term memory [20]. However, some studies suggest that RAN is independent of phonological processing and can, itself, account for variance in reading. This implies that a naming deficit is directly related to orthographic processing- if letters are recognized at a slower rate, letter representations of words are not activated with sufficient speed to create a strong trace of common orthographic features [21]. Further support for this view is found in research that confirms that later in reading skill development, the role of non-alphanumeric RAN diminishes, while that of alphanumeric RAN (letters and digits) increases and becomes the sole predictor of reading at this stage [22]. From a global perspective, this naming speed deficit seems to be more prominent than the phonological deficit, and this appears to be true in both transparent orthographies like Spanish, Finnish, and German, as well as in entirely different and diverse orthographies, such as Hebrew, Chinese, and Japanese [23].

3. A review of international studies and phonological processing/speed

International researchers have investigated many of the most important factors identified in fluent reading. In Dutch, Vaessen and Blomert found that RAN contributed uniquely and substantially to the development of word reading fluency from grade 1 to grade 6 in primary school students [24], and when both accuracy and speed measures were considered in French, readers with dyslexia displayed deficiency in word-level reading skills [25]. A similar speed deficit of lexical and sub-lexical reading was also suggested by findings in French dyslexic children. The suggestion here being that the sub-lexical route shares with the lexical one the initial processing of the letter string, but then the lexical processing applies grapheme-phoneme rules in a serial mode [26]. This deficiency in sub-lexical processing is also a crucial feature in American dyslexic definitions and treatment, a language system known for its irregular words and "exceptions to the rule".

Researchers have proposed that between English and German dyslexic children with the same underlying phonological processing deficit, the English children show more severe reading impairment because of differences in orthographic consistency [27]. Mann and Wimmer [28] assessed readers in English and German at the end of kindergarten, and regression analyses showed that the only significant predictor of reading accuracy and speed in English was phonological awareness. Initial studies in German children found few problems with accuracy after the first year of instruction in contrast to English-based research and led to a German-English dyslexia comparison [27]. However, the reading fluency deficit of German dyslexic readers (found for all types of reading tasks) was found to be highly persistent [29] and hard to remediate [30].

Extensive research with German and Italian dyslexic children found reduced reading fluency as the main dyslexic impairment [6, 31]. Impairment on tasks that require implicit phonological processing, such as those evaluating verbal short-term memory, has been identified most clearly in transparent orthographies such as Italian and German [32]. Italian is a relatively shallow orthography, characterized by a high consistency of grapheme-phoneme correspondences and a simple syllabic structure. Also there are few irregular words and non-homographic homophones [15]. In spite of this regular orthography, Italian children with Developmental Dyslexia still present with a relevant difficulty which is primarily a deficit in reading speed [33] markedly affected by stimulus length [34]. Tobia and Marzocchi worked to define the cognitive profile of Italian children with Developmental Dyslexia. They found that 43.7% of children with DD had a profile that included deficits in both verbal and nonverbal domains. Some measures (visual search, syllable blending, and syllable deletion) were not significantly different among the three groups: dyslexic children, typically developing children of the same age (CA) and a control group of younger children equated for reading ability. Phoneme blending was the only variable that showed a large effect size [35].

The viability of accuracy/fluency-based typology of reading impairments has been investigated in Hebrew by Shany and Share [2]. Using a full battery of behavioral assessments including "pointed texts" (with all diacritical vowel markings included) and "unpointed texts" (with partial vowel markings included), these researchers found clear processing differences between the performances of students identified as rate-disabled and those identified as accuracy-disabled. Especially for word reading, the doubly-disabled subgroup of students was the most severely incapacitated with the lowest accuracy and reading rates.

The Korean handwriting system is an "alpha-syllabic" orthography, called Hangul. There are 24 graphemes, 14 are consonants and 10 are basic vowels. Hangul graphemes consistently represent sounds with a one-to-one correspondence and are combined in a limited number of patterns [36]. In a study using Hangul, researchers investigated the association of RAN and regular/irregular words in 4- and 5-year-old Korean children and found that RAN was uniquely associated with reading ability of both regular and irregular words [37]. Other research examined the cognitive abilities that predict reading and spelling performance in Korean children in Grades 1–4. Park and Uno [36] found that the contribution of phonological awareness to Hangul reading accuracy appears to occur only during the first 2 years of schooling, and RAN speed significantly predicted word-reading accuracy only in Grade 1. Further, the results of path analysis revealed that receptive vocabulary contributed exclusively and substantially to Hangul word-reading accuracy in Grades 1–4. This is unusual in light of the accepted idea that vocabulary plays a more important role in reading in less consistent orthographies [17]. Park and Uno argue that these results may be due to characteristics of the Hangul writing system that support the decoding of two-syllable words based on partial decoding and knowledge of the phonological and lexical aspects of a known, corresponding spoken word. In this case, the strategies needed to read accurately and with speed in Hangul differ with expertise and reading experience. A recent cross-language investigation measured reading performance (both reading accuracy and fluency), phonological short-term memory, RAN, receptive vocabulary and non-verbal intelligence in grade 2 children in five European countries (Finland, France, Hungary, Netherlands, and Portugal). While it is often proposed that extensive familiarity with the words of a language affects reading performance, the results here suggest that vocabulary was not a unique predictor of reading accuracy and fluency in these languages, except for Finnish [38].

In conclusion, phonological awareness represents the main predictive factor in normal and disabled readers of different languages. However, it may be less relevant in consistent orthographies, especially for reading accuracy where language –specific patterns appear to exist [39]. Research in German [40], Dutch [41], Norwegian [42], Italian [33], Greek [43], Finnish [44], Hungarian [45], and Hebrew [46], shows that most dyslexics in these languages attain high levels of reading accuracy but remain slow. It is possible that orthographies that are relatively regular in their letter-sound correspondences such as the Arabic require rapid development of the "direct access route". Perhaps it is only with increasing practice that improvements in efficiency lead to the reliable use of "direct access processes". Consequently, it is unclear whether the sub-lexical route accesses semantics after the phonology is assembled, and it is still debated whether direct visual access can occur without phonological mediation [47]. See **Table 1** for a time-ordered summary of the international studies cited regarding phonological processing.

Researchers	National origin of subjects	Year	Subjects- age or grade	Major findings
Wimmer	Germany	1993	Grades 2, 3, 4	German dyslexics attain high levels of reading accuracy but remain slow in processing speed.
Yap, Van der Leij	Netherlands	1993	Mean age: 10.2 years	Dutch dyslexics attain high levels of reading accuracy but remain slow in processing speed.
Bjaalid, Hoien, Lundberg	Norway	1996	Grade 3	Norwegian dyslexics attain high levels of reading accuracy but remain slow in processing speed.
Breznitz	Israel	1997	Normal mean age: 6.9 years; Dyslexic: 9.1 years	Hebrew dyslexics attain high levels of reading accuracy but remain slow in processing speed.
Landerl, Wimmer, Frith	Germany, England	1997	8 year olds	English children seem more impaired because of orthographic differences; German children had few problems with accuracy after the first year of instruction.

Researchers	National origin of subjects	Year	Subjects- age or grade	Major findings
Wimmer, Mayringer, Landerl	Germany, Italy	1998	Beginning Gr. 1 and End Gr. 2	Impairment on verbal short-term memory has been identified most clearly in transparent orthographies.
Porpodas	Greece	1999	Grade 1	Greek dyslexics attain high levels of reading accuracy but remain slow in processing speed.
Zoccolotti, De Luca, Di Pace, Judica, Orlandi, et al.	Italy	1999	11–15 years old	Italian children with DD demonstrate primarily a deficit in reading speed.
De Luca, Borrelli, Judica, Spinelli, Zoccolotti	Germany, Italy	2002	11–16 years old	Reduced reading fluency is the main impairment in German and Italian dyslexic children.
Mann, Wimmer	Germany, England	2002	End of Kindergarten	Phonological awareness was the only significant predictor of reading accuracy and speed in English students.
Hutzler, Wimmer	Germany, Italy	2004	13 yr. olds	Reduced reading fluency is the main impairment in German and Italian dyslexic children.
Thaler, Ebner, Wimmer, Landerl	Germany	2004	8–11 years old	Reading fluency deficit in German Dyslexic readers is hard to remediate.
Zoccolotti, De Luca, Di Pace, Gasperini, Judica, et al.	Italy	2005	Grades 1, 2, 3	Reading speed deficits in Italian children with DD are markedly affected by stimulus length.
Puolakanaho, Ahonen, Aro, Eklund, Leppanen, et al.	Finland	2007	3.5, 4.5, and 5.5 years old	Finnish dyslexics attain high levels of reading accuracy but remain slow in processing speed.
Cho, Mcbride-Chang, Park	Korea	2008	4 and 5 yr. olds	RAN was uniquely associated with reading ability of both regular and irregular words.
Georgiou, Parrila, Papadopoulos		2008	Grades 1 and 2	Phonological awareness may be less relevant in consistent orthographies.
Landerl, Wimmer	Germany	2008	Gr. 1, 4, 8	Reading fluency deficit in German dyslexic readers is highly persistent.
Vaessen, Blomert	Netherlands	2010	Grade 1–6	RAN contributed uniquely and substantially to word reading fluency.
Ziegler, Bertrand, Tóth, Csépe, Reis, et al.	Finland, France, Hungary, Portugal, Netherlands	2010	Grade 2	Vocabulary was not a significant predictor of reading accuracy and fluency in these languages, except for Finnish.

Researchers	National origin of subjects	Year	Subjects- age or grade	Major findings
Shany, Share	Israel	2011	Grades 2, 4, 6	There are processing differences between rate-disabled and accuracy-disabled readers; the doubly-disabled readers had the lowest accuracy and reading rates.
Sprenger-Charolles	France, Spain, England	2011	7 yr. olds	French dyslexics were weak in word reading when both accuracy and speed were measured.
Csépe, Honbolygó, Paavo, Leppänen	Hungary	2012	Grades 2–4	Hungarian dyslexics attain high levels of reading accuracy but remain slow in processing speed.
Tobia, Marzocchi	Italy	2014	DD grp. Mean age: 9.76 years; Control grp. 9.82 years; RA grp. 7.38 years	Results show that 43.7% of Italian children with DD showed deficits in both verbal and nonverbal domains; phoneme blending was the only variable that predicted reading disability.
Park, Uno	Korea	2015	Grades 1–4	RAN speed significantly predicted word-reading accuracy only in Grade 1; receptive vocabulary contributed exclusively and significantly to word reading accuracy.

Table 1.
International studies of phonological processing in time order.

4. A review of international studies and visual processing

An interesting element of learning to read in a regular orthography is the relative ease of attaining high levels of accuracy. Correct reading in transparent orthographies is already at ceiling level after the first year of formal instruction [5, 17]. The advantage of regular orthography was further documented in studies comparing a substantial number of regular European writing systems with English [5, 48]. Due to the transparency of the language system, visual processing deficits are often found to contribute to dyslexia. In a Norwegian study, Talcott et al. demonstrated the presence of visual processing deficits characteristic of poor readers in a sample of poor readers [49]. Finnish is one of the most regular alphabetic orthographies and dyslexia primarily means slow dysfluent reading, however a major dysfunction of the occipito-temporal reading circuit is suggested by a series of MEG studies with Finnish dyslexic adults [50]. A dysfunction of left occipito-temporal reading areas was also found in the cross-linguistic PET study by Paulesu et al. [51] which included dyslexic adult readers from the regular Italian orthography and from less regular orthographies of French and English. There is also a good deal of evidence that children with Developmental Dyslexia also experience difficulties in visuo-attentional tasks [52], such as visual search [53], visual recognition [54], and low-level (occurring within the first 300 milliseconds of visual analysis) visual information processing [55]. Thai researchers examined the performance of good and poor 10 year-old Thai readers on visual processing and reading accuracy tests and found a difference between the good and poor Thai readers in their performance on visual processing tests [56].

Schiff et al., [57] examined the effects of orthographic transparency on the reading ability of fourth-grade children with dyslexia on two Hebrew scripts. In addition to documenting reading accuracy and speed, this study also investigated the role of vowelization in the reading ability of un-vowelized script among readers with dyslexia. These results showed that fourth-grade children with dyslexia read the vowelized script with less accuracy than that found in typically developing second-graders. Also, the children with dyslexia demonstrated no significant differences in the reading accuracy or speed between the vowelized and unvowelized scripts. However, for these readers with dyslexia, accuracy in reading both vowelized and un-vowelized words mediated the reading speed of un-vowelized scripts. These findings underscore the idea that if grapheme-phoneme conversion skills are flawed in Hebrew children with dyslexia, they are unable to use the vowelized script as a self-teaching mechanism for acquiring an autonomous orthographic lexicon that would enable future word recognition.

The hypothesis of poor phonological-orthographic integration suggests impaired neural connectivity between regions engaged by orthographic processes and regions engaged in phonological processes [58]. There are first reports suggesting abnormalities of the left-hemisphere tracts that connect occipito-temporal brain regions engaged by visual-orthographic processes with temporo-parietal and the left inferior frontal areas engaged by phonological processes [59]. Functional imaging findings- some with German dyslexic readers -show reduced reading related activation in a left ventral occipito-temporal brain region, which is assumed to function as an interface between high-level visual orthographic codes and phonology and meaning. As expected, dysfluent readers exhibited underactivation of the left occipito-temporal region of interest-ROI (engaged by fast word processing) and increased activation of the left inferior frontal ROI (engaged by phonological decoding) [60]. Voxel-based analysis showed that for fluent readers, extended activations were found in the left temporal cortex mainly along the superior temporal sulcus and in left inferior frontal and precentral regions. The left temporal activation extended into the supramarginal gyrus and inferior occipito-temporal cortex. More issues regarding neural connectivity will be investigated in depth later.

A fascinating example of an opaque and complex orthographic system used in India is found in the Urdu language system. There are 38 letters with no vowel letters, and diacritics, which serve as vowel markings in its script, are omitted. The graphemic system called Nastaliq is cursive, and is characterized by many to one mappings between graphic symbols and sounds. Further, the same letter is written differently in different positions in a word, [61] greatly increasing the possible variations of each letter. Most Indian children speak Punjabi as their first language, but Urdu is the national language and the language of the media. It is the medium of instruction at schools, and another first language for some children, depending on the social class. In all Pakistani schools, English is taught and evaluated as a compulsory subject from grade 1, but in Urdu medium schools, all subjects are taught in Urdu, and English is taught as a subject, and in English medium schools, all subjects are taught in English, and Urdu is taught as a subject. There are clearly differences in the instruction and informal practice of reading and writing the Urdu language in different settings. For both the control group and the reading disability group, both RAN letters and RAN digits significantly predicted fluency with RAN letters being the stronger predictor. For the control group, non-word reading was the most significant predictor of accuracy and RAN letters was the other significant predictor. For the reading disability group, only RAN letters predicted accuracy [61]. So even in a visually complicated, reading-in-a-second (or third) language, rapid naming is shown to be an important predictor of reading accuracy. However, the most compelling issue regarding fluency around the world may be that in spite of different orthographies and language regularities, commonly-used instructional interventions still do not result in lasting remediation for the majority of this population. See **Table 2** for a time-ordered summary of the international studies cited regarding orthographic processing.

Researchers	National origin of subjects	Year	Subjects	Major Findings
Slaghuis, Lovegrove	Australia	1987	13 year olds	Children with DD show difficulties with low-level visual information processing.
Eden, Vanmeter, Rumsey, Maisog, Woods, et al.	United States	1996	Adult men	Men with DD show difficulties with visuo-attentional tasks.
Paulesu, Demonet, Fazio, Mccrory, Chanoine, et al.	England, France, Italy	2001	Dyslexic adults	In a cross-linguistic PET study, a dysfunction of left occipito-temporal reading areas was found.
Seymour, Aro, Erskine	Denmark, England, Finland, France, Germany, Greece, Iceland, Italy, Netherlands, Norway, Portugal, Spain, Sweden	2003	6, 7, 8, yr. olds	Reading accuracy in transparent orthographies is at ceiling level after the first year of instruction.
Talcott, Gram, van Ingelghem, Witton, Stein, et al.	Norway	2003	12, 13, 14 yr. olds	Visual processing deficits were characteristic of poor readers.
Kim, Davis, Burnham, Luksaneeyanawin	Thailand	2004	10-year old children	There is a difference in good and poor Thai readers in their performance on visual processing tests.
Salmelin, Helenius	Finland	2004	Dyslexic adults	MEG studies reveal a major dysfunction of the occipito-temporal reading circuit
Deutsch, Dougherty, Bammer, Siok, Gabrieli, et al.	United States	2005	7–13 year olds	First reports suggesting abnormalities of the left-hemisphere tracts that connect occipito-temporal brain regions with temporo-parietal and left inferior frontal areas.
Kronbichler, Hutzler, Staffen, Mair, Ladurner, et al.	Germany	2006	14–16 year olds	Dysfluent readers showed underactivation of the left occipito-temporal region and increased activation in a left inferior frontal region.
Geiger, Cattaneo, Galli, Pozzoli, Lorusso, et al.	Italy	2008	9–13 year olds	Children with DD show difficulties with visual recognition.
Vidyasagar, Pammer	Australia	2010	7–12 year olds	Children with DD show difficulties with visual search.
Schiff, Katzir, Shoshan	Israel	2013	Grade 4	There were no significant differences in reading accuracy or speed in dyslexic readers regardless of the text (vowelized or un-vowelized).

Table 2.
International studies of orthographic processing in time order.

5. The development of fluency in English

The American focus on the development of reading proficiency has been far-ranging and often perplexing, perhaps due to the intricacies of the English language. It has been considered that the cognitive processes underpinning reading ability may be differently involved in producing the symptoms of Developmental Dyslexia, depending on orthographic transparency [29]. Converging data from a variety of neurobiological investigations, but especially from functional magnetic resonance imaging, support the current belief that there are differences in the temporo-parieto-occipital brain regions between dyslexic and nonimpaired readers. Goswami [62] found that analysis of results from different technologies, including PET, fMRI, MEG, and EEG using different research questions, consistently show that children with Developmental Dyslexia display hypoactivation of crucial parts of the network of areas involved in word recognition and an atypical pattern of continuing right hemisphere involvement.

The neurobiological origins of fluency can actually be seen in the early work of physiologist, Donald Hebb. In 1950, he proposed the concept of unitization when he observed patterns of cells in the visual cortex activating together after multiple exposures to novel visual stimuli [63]. LaBerge and Samuels went on to apply this idea to more complex visual levels such as familiar letter patterns, and in other modalities such as phonological representations. They focused on the automaticity of processing that decreases response time in learning and reading and is believed to increase the neurological resources allocated to comprehension [64]. American educators have historically used fluency as a measure of reading performance and a precursor of superior comprehension, but continue to fail in developing instructional exercises that improve reading speed, especially for those with specific reading disabilities. The expectation is that students will read fluently as a function of age and experience. Oral reading inventories and running records of reading performance commonly measure fluency as the rate and accuracy of oral reading and ignore the other aspects of fluency, particularly the contributions of lower level subskills: graphological features of letters, orthographic regularities of letter combinations, the semantic features of words, and the semantic-syntactic constraints of word sequences.

Ultimately, Kame'enui, Simmons, Good, and Harn suggested a developmental conceptualization of fluency that included the building of proficiency in foundational component skills of reading, effectively merging the influences of skill development with processing speed and accuracy into a continuum of reading proficiency [65]. It is this continuum that Wolf and Katzir-Cohen refer to in their comprehensive definition of fluency:

"In its beginnings, reading fluency is the product of the initial development of accuracy and the subsequent development of automaticity in underlying sublexical process, lexical processes, and their integration in single-word reading and connected text. These include perceptual, phonological, orthographic, and morphological processes at the letter, letter-pattern, and word levels, as well as semantic and syntactic processes at the word level and the connected text level. After it is fully developed, reading fluency refers to a level of accuracy and rate where decoding is relatively effortless; where oral reading is smooth and accurate with correct prosody; and where attention can be allocated to comprehension." [66]

Since the development of fluency is founded in every process and skill used in reading, Kame'enui [67] advises that it also requires an increase in proficiency and speed in every underlying component. It seems obvious that failure to acquire these processes and skills would result in critical and persistent reading disabilities.

Researchers have been diligent to identify the progressive neurodevelopment of those underlying processes. It is clear that Frith's 1997 phonological deficit hypothesis which suggests that Developmental Dyslexia results from an underlying phonological impairment, and accounts for a wide range of behavioral symptoms associated with dyslexia, especially lexical retrieval and verbal short-term memory, has been thoroughly validated [68].

Further, the issue of general intellectual ability has been explored with regard to phonological processing. Although the 2004 reauthorization of the U.S.'s Individuals with Disabilities Act mandates that states can no longer require school districts to use IQ tests to identify individuals with learning disabilities [69], the majority of schools and school psychologists still rely on the discrepancy between reading achievement and IQ to define dyslexia [70]: requiring that reading skill should be significantly below the level expected given an individual's IQ. Tanaka et al. used fMRI, univariate, and multivariate pattern analysis to observe whether differences in brain activation during phonological processing that are characteristic of readers with dyslexia were the same or different in dyslexic children with poor reading ability who had high IQ scores (discrepant readers) and in dyslexic children with poor reading ability who had low IQ scores (non-discrepant readers) as compared to the phonological processing of typically developing readers [71]. The results show that discrepant and non-discrepant poor readers exhibited similar patterns of reduced activation in brain areas such as left parieto-temporal and occipito-temporal regions; there were no reliable functional brain differences between the two types of poor readers. The validity of the discrepancy definition of dyslexia is called into question. Even though the discrepancy criterion may be intuitively appealing, its strict application would deprive non-discrepant children of the educational interventions that could promote their advancement in reading.

American researchers have also found distinctions in the use of RAN for identifying impaired processing. Using multi-variant analysis of the results of a battery of reading skills measures of 123 dyslexic 2nd and 3rd graders, Katzir et al. found that rapid naming, orthographic pattern recognition, and word reading fluency moderately predicted rate, accuracy, and comprehension of connected-text reading, while phonological awareness contributed only to the comprehension dimension of connected-text reading [72]. The unanticipated result that rapid naming was more related to reading speed than phonological awareness may help explain the limited success of phonology-based reading intervention programs for achieving improvements in fluency and comprehension.

6. Intervention studies impacting English

Researchers in the U.S. have also investigated the effects of focused instruction and other interventions. Several post-intervention studies show different patterns of activation in the reading networks, evidence of the strength of experimental results in suggesting effective neurobiologically-based remedial instructional practices. Shaywitz et al. found increased LH activation of the inferior frontal gyrus (IFG) and the middle temporal gyrus only in children with the characteristics of dyslexia who participated in daily tutoring of the alphabetic principle and phonological processing and not in those children who participated in a variety of common reading interventions exclusive of explicit phonology [73]. Their longitudinal data also indicated a continuation of correct activation patterns 1 year past, suggesting the durable nature of the processing change. Similarly, Simos, Breier, Fletcher, Bergman, and Papanicolaou using MSI found that after 80 hours of intensive phonological intervention, dyslexic children showed a dramatic increase in the activation of left temporo-parietal regions, predominately in the left posterior superior temporal gyrus (STG), the network that supports grapheme-phoneme recoding in typical developing readers. However, even after intervention, neural activity was delayed in the dyslexic children relative to the controls (837 ms on average for dyslexics and 600 ms for controls), indicating that even with intensive phonological remediation, dyslexic children are slower to achieve the same reading fluency shown by non-dyslexic children. Further, high-risk children, who were nonresponsive to the phonological remediation package that was being offered, were distinct in showing earlier onset of activity in IFG compared to the temporo-parietal regions [74]. This would indicate a persistent processing anomaly that influences ineffective decoding as well as decreased processing speed.

However, it is the work of Dutch and Italian researchers that provided the foundation for a fluency intervention that appears to address the processing anomalies that are prevalent in American dyslexics. Employing the commonly accepted differences in the hemispheric contributions in learning to read, Bakker and Vinke identified Dutch children with dyslexia as L-dyslexics or P-dyslexics based on oral reading error analysis, the distribution of brain responses, and other behavioral measures [75]. They proposed that L-dyslexics are insensitive to the perceptual features of text because they predominately developed left hemisphere strategies from the very onset of learning to read. Behaviorally, L-dyslexics exhibit a hurried and inaccurate style of reading with many word substitution errors. Conversely, P-dyslexics are overly sensitive to perceptual features of the text because they began the learning-to-read process in the right hemisphere, but never advanced from there. These P-dyslexics read slowly with a fragmented style. Bakker and Vinke hypothesized that since L-type dyslexics had trouble using right hemispheric strategies during reading, they might profit from specific stimulation of the right hemisphere and the opposite for P-dyslexics: they had not naturally shifted to left hemisphere processing and so would benefit from specific stimulation of the left hemisphere [75].

As a general rule, specific stimulation of a hemisphere (HSS) can be achieved by the lateral presentation of a stimulus (reading material) in the left visual field or to the fingers of the left hand in L-dyslexics, and in the right visual field or to the fingers of the right hand in P-dyslexics. Bakker and Vinke actually treated the children with a wooden tactile training box, in which the child would place their target arm through a hole in the side and manipulate plastic letters in grooves out of sight. L-type children were given regularly-formed concrete words to configure and trace with their left hand, to stimulate the right hemisphere. P-type children were given difficult-to-visualize abstract words to configure and trace with their right hand, to stimulate the left hemisphere. The results indicated that P-dyslexics showed a decrease in sound/symbol errors on both word and text reading, while L-dyslexics decreased substantive errors only on text reading [75]. In spite of several limitations in their methodology and intervention, the positive effects of even motor stimulation to the less activated hemisphere on reading performance are encouraging. Further, these findings imply that the dyslexia sub-typing procedures appear to be valid techniques for matching reading interventions to brain processing systems.

Based on the potency of these theoretical and neurobiological foundations, Lorusso, Facoetti, Paganoni, Pezzani, and Molteni achieved much stronger results in a study of Italian impaired readers employing computer technology. These researchers implemented the sub-typing of dyslexic students used by Bakker and Vinke, and added M- type dyslexia: a mixed type demonstrating both slow and inaccurate reading, indicating impaired processing in both hemispheres [76]. Their new technology included a modified version of a computerized system for visual hemisphere-specific stimulation (VHSS), "FlashWord" [77]. After 1440 minutes (24 h) of intervention, Lorusso et al. applied only behavioral measures and found that all students with the characteristics of dyslexia, regardless of their sub-type, improved not only in accuracy and fluency as compared to non-impaired controls, but also showed gains in spelling, memory, and general processing speed. Further, the dyslexic students gained 0.33 syllables / second more in reading speed over the same period of time than their non-impaired controls [76]. These extraordinary results suggest that requiring very fast processing of the presented visual stimuli in a targeted brain hemisphere may produce a greater degree of automatisation of the component processes. It is this automatisation of the underlying lexical and sublexical processes that Wolfe and Katzir-Cohen validate as critical influences on fluent reading of connected text in their comprehensive definition of fluency [66].

7. VHSS intervention in English

Subsequent research using FlashWord in English with American students has built on the successes in Dutch and Italian. Koen et al. used fMRI technology to localize brain activity before and after VHSS training in students who qualified with the characteristics of developmental dyslexia. This research was designed to test the hypothesis that subtyping students with the characteristics of dyslexia based on their reading behaviors as Bakker proposed, and administering VHSS intervention based on those subtypes (FlashWord-modified and in English), would improve fluency performance across dyslexia sub-types more effectively than other currently used reading fluency programs. Secondarily, the location and level of activation differences from pre-intervention and post-intervention scans were analyzed for evidence of developing automaticity in regions of interest [78].

FlashWord, Ver. 2.2, written by Franco Fabbro and Cristina Masutto (copyright, 1995–2004 by Editrice TecnoScuola) is a computer program that uses a game-format to present words or phrases in the right or left visual hemi-field at increasingly rapid rates. According to their dyslexia sub-type, each student sees the words (or phrases) projected on either the right or left side of the computer screen, stimulating either the right or left visual field and the opposite brain hemisphere. Ocular fixation is confirmed by directing the child to watch a luminous dot oscillating up and down on the screen at an adjustable speed. A word is revealed only when the child clicks the mouse exactly when the dot is crossing the central target. This ensures visual attention to the stimulus. The child's task is to read the words as they are flashed on the screen in ever shortening durations. Reading rates of 250–100 ms for single words are generally considered to reflect "emerging fluency" [75]. For this study, students repeated all of the lessons in their assigned program (34 for the LH program and 27 for the RH program) at their own speed, matching the Italian students in total time spent: 1440 minutes (or 24 hours) total.

This fMRI experiment used a mixed design, in that the events of interest (Word Pair analysis) are randomized with perceptual controls (Letter Match analysis) to provide robust event-related activation maps and estimates of hemodynamic response. The Letter Match task demands that the child decide whether two letter strings (e.g., szpy and sxpy), printed in all black letters and shown simultaneously one above the other, match exactly. The length of the letter strings is comparable to the length of the pseudo-words used in the phonological analysis task. As this is the control task, attention to all letter positions is necessary but the assignment of speech sounds to letters is not. For the phonological analysis task, the Word Pairs were two decodable non-words printed in black, also presented visually, one above the other. Each word contained a letter, or group of letters, printed in pink. The child was instructed to press the button "Yes", if the pink letter(s) in the top word could stand for the same sound as the pink letter(s) in the bottom word, and to press a different button "No", if the pink letters represent different sounds.

Among other statistical procedures, the results of 1440 minutes of intervention measured in milliseconds and representing a change in speed of processing was used as a measure of achieved fluency in the Intervention group only. This sub-grouping was necessary because three individuals in the Intervention group did not achieve fluent processing with the FastWord program. This evidence of processing change was analyzed by means of a two-way mixed design ANOVA having two levels of reading fluency scores (pre- and post-intervention) as a within-subjects factor and two levels of fluency: those students ($N = 6$) who reached levels of emerging fluency, 100 ms or less, and those ($N = 3$) who did not, as a between-subjects factor. The between-subjects main effect of the fluency rate achieved during intervention was significant, $F(1,8) = 5.38$, $p = .05$, indicating significant differences between the students who achieved fluent processing and those who did not [78].

The fMRI results were remarkable for their corroboration of brain activations found during tasks requiring phoneme analysis. This analysis focused on three Regions of Interest (ROIs) within the core sub-systems supporting the processing of written language in normal readers: the left hemisphere (LH) superior temporal gyrus (STG) in the inferior parietal lobule within the temporoparietal system associated with word meaning; the posterior aspect of the inferior frontal gyrus (IFG) within the anterior system associated with sound/symbol associations; and the LH inferior occipito-temporal/fusiform area (VWFA) within the ventral system associated with quick recall of high frequency words first documented by Shaywitz et al. [73]. It was hypothesized that achieving fluency in reading will involve automaticity within each of these ROIs and that the brain activation maps of phonological processing of Word Pairs greater than perceptual control of Letter Match condition would show changes in activation patterns. Through comparisons of pre-intervention processing and post-intervention processing, there are clearly subjects who demonstrate much more focused activation bilaterally in the temporal regions around the STG and Postcentral Gyrus with very little activation in the visual word form area (VWFA) in the LH occipital lobe, and others who show an increase in left hemisphere activation around the IFG and VWFA [78].

Using a clustering threshold of five voxels, a sample of the activation locations were found post-intervention in the condition of Word Pairs over Letter Match in a fluent subject. **Table 3** contains a partial list of left hemisphere only activation sites, noting the location, relative size, and maximum recorded t-score.

These data confirm some anticipated activation areas with sizeable groups of voxels contributing and some remarkable lack of activation within the ROIs studied. The largest activated cluster in the IFG ROI is the Inferior Frontal Gyrus (1.52), but activation in the STG (3.10), and Brodmann areas 41 (3.17) and 42 (3.94) is much stronger. This could indicate that most of the processing in this region involved sound/symbol associations with support in the primary and auditory association cortex. The weak activation in the IFG, which supports the encoding of phonological features, could mean that less effort was required to accomplish the phonological analysis task by this subject.

The largest activated cluster in the STG ROI is the STG (2.56), but again, other areas show stronger levels of stimulation. The Postcentral Gyrus activation (3.87) is odd in that this area is the primary somatosensory cortex receiving all sensory input, especially touch. However, except for the pressing of the response button, there was no variation in the motor demands of the scanner task that would explain activation in this area. The activation found in Brodmann areas 13 (3.08) and 40

Structure	x	y	z	Cluster size	Max t score
ROI-IFG					
LH inferior frontal gyrus	−48	24	12	523	1.52
LH superior temporal gyrus	−60	−28	12	352	3.10
LH Brodmann area 41	−56	−20	12	147	3.71
LH insula	−36	−16	12	119	1.97
LH Brodmann area 42	−60	−20	−12	114	3.94
LH Brodmann area 13	−40	−16	12	73	1.93
LH precentral gyrus	−56	−8	12	67	1.66
ROI-STG					
LH superior temporal gyrus	−40	−40	16	233	2.56
LH angular gyrus	−52	−64	36	86	2.46
LH insula	−42	−16	16	68	2.21
LH postcentral gyrus	−52	−31	52	33	3.87
LH Brodmann area 13	−44	−16	16	29	3.08
LH inferior parietal lobule	−52	−36	28	26	2.74
ROI-VWFA					
LH sub-gyral	−36	−4	−32	30	1.54
LH middle temporal gyrus	−40	0	−32	19	1.42
LH Brodmann area 20	−44	−8	−32	7	1.80
LH Brodmann area 21	−40	−4	−32	5	2.05
LH Brodmann area 35	−24	−16	−32	5	2.01
LH fusiform (aal)	−28	−24	−32	5	3.06

Table 3.
Post-intervention activation locations in a fluent subject.

(3.16) makes sense in that area 40 is part of Wernicke's Gyrus where sound/symbol associations are refined and area 13 is a bridge between lateral and medial layers. The Postcentral activation could be evidence of compensatory systems being used for phonological analysis in immature processing systems.

The largest activation in the VWFA ROI is found in the smallest clusters detected. The Brodmann areas 21 (2.05) and 35 (2.01) appear to support automatic processing through their connection to Middle Temporal Gyrus, believed to access word meaning, and the perirhinal cortex, critical to memory. The left aspect of the Fusiform Gyrus shows the strongest activation (3.06) as would be expected if automatic retrieval of letter patterns was triggered [78]. So taken together, the activation locations identified in the subjects of this study, generally follow activation patterns found in the literature. Shaywitz et al. found that activation in the left occipito-temporal cortex increases with reading skill [79].

Even more unexpected, was the finding that only 1440 minutes of intervention resulted in increases in the reading speed of connected text for many subjects. Since the training mostly involved single word reading and some phrases, it was not anticipated that the intervention would make any difference in the reading of longer passages of connected text. However, this was found to be false. Six of the nine students in the Intervention Group who achieved levels of automatic

Intervention Group (N = 9)			Delayed Intervention Group (N = 6)		
Pre-intervention reading fluency range (average)	Post-intervention reading fluency range (average)	Net gain	Pre-intervention reading fluency range (average)	Post-intervention reading fluency range (average)	Net gain
40–115 wpm (78 wpm)	51–131 wpm (90 wpm)	11.9 wpm	24–128 wpm (77 wpm)	50–120 wpm (85 wpm)	7.3

Table 4.
Summary of behavioral results.

processing (<100 ms) in either the left- or right visual hemi-field, also increased their reading rate by an average of 20 wpm [78]. See **Table 4**.

There is considerable evidence that different students responded to the intervention differently. Those students who only displayed phonics-based errors in reading connected text and worked for the entire intervention time in the LH Program seemed to make the most substantial increases in both processing and reading speed. Only one student who demonstrated meaning-based errors and used the RH Program exclusively showed faster processing during intervention. The students who displayed both types of errors and split their time between programs made the least amount of progress; two reached fluency in the LH Program, but not in the RH Program. It is suggested that continued work with the intervention program could achieve the desired level of automaticity and that strengthening processing in the right hemisphere is inherently more difficult than strengthening the left hemisphere [78].

Wolf cautions that another source of reading disability could be an impediment in the circuit connections among the brain structures, stressing the importance of understanding the connectivity among the various regions instrumental to reading performance. She proposed at least three forms of disconnections which are consistently studied: between the frontal and posterior language regions based on under-activity in the connecting insula; and between the occipital-temporal region or the left angular gyrus region; and frontal areas in the left hemisphere. She suggests that children with dyslexia use an altogether different reading circuitry. Instead of a progressive disentanglement of the right hemisphere's larger visual recognition system in reading words and an increasing engagement of left hemisphere's frontal, temporal, and occipital-temporal regions, they used more frontal regions, showed less activity in the left-hemisphere angular gyrus, and created potentially compensatory "auxillary" right-hemisphere regions which performed functions usually handled by more efficient left-hemisphere areas [14]. The fMRI results from this study underscore Wolf's proposal. It may be that much of the diffuse frontal activation that was observed in many pre-intervention scans and some post-intervention scans of nonfluent subjects is evidence of these compensatory "auxillary" strategies. It may be that in older readers who have over time consolidated less efficient pathways for reading, more exposure is required for specific hemispheric stimulation (intervention) to supplant frontal and right hemisphere functions with effective left hemisphere processing.

8. Case studies OF VHSS intervention

Subject 1, coded MC, was one of the students who reached very fast processing speeds during the intervention using the left hemisphere program. The pre-intervention scan showed mostly diffuse activation in the right hemisphere occipital-parietal areas. Based on all phonetic reading errors in the pre-intervention fluency measure, this student was labeled a "P-type" and assigned the LH intervention program. MC was a very willing subject and engaged with the program easily. After progressing through the LH program (34 lessons) nearly six times during the 1440 minutes of training, the fastest processing was 80 ms with 100% accuracy. This student also achieved fluent processing rather quickly on the thirteenth day of treatment. MC gained 26 wpm on the final fluency measure. Analyzing this subject's scanner data, there was an almost perfect performance when processing the letter matches: 98% accuracy during Scan 1 and 89% accuracy during Scan 2. MC's analysis of phonemic elements improved from Scan 1–2. During Scan 1, 54% of the word pairs were correctly identified and 70% were right in Scan 2. Overall this subject demonstrated a 5% improvement in fast decoding skills. The post-intervention scan shows much more focused activation bilaterally in the temporal regions around the superior temporal gyrus and postcentral gyrus, and there is very little activation in the VWFA in the LH occipital lobe [78].

Subject 2, coded PE, was one of the students who achieved processing speeds that approached fluency using the left hemisphere program. The pre-intervention scan showed a lot of bilateral frontal activation and more RH activation than LH activation in the occipital areas. Five out of six reading errors were phonics-based, so this student was labeled "P-type" and assigned the LH program. PE completed the LH program six times during 1440 minutes of treatment, but there were only 24 lessons included because some of the orthographic patterns were not taught at this reading level. This student was one of the younger participants in the study and only reached levels of fluent processing for words, not for phrases. PE's fastest processing score was 125 ms with 83% accuracy and during post-intervention fluency measures, reading speed was increased by 11 wpm. Analyzing the scanner data, there is evidence of significant learning, perhaps due to the young age and the nature of reading instruction in the lower grades. PE showed a lot of confusion when analyzing the letter strings: only 49% were judged correctly in Scan 1 and 57% in Scan 2. Growth in decoding skills is evident in the correct identification of the word pairs: 45% during Scan 1 and 62% during Scan 2. Overall, this subject demonstrated a 13% improvement in fast visual processing. The post-intervention scan indicates an increase in left hemisphere activation around the inferior frontal gyrus and VWFA [78].

So if the focus is on automatic word retrieval, the Visual Word Form Area, has to be a region of exceptional interest. There remains much to understand regarding the activation of the Visual Word Form Area in the left fusiform gyrus and its relationship to the development of fluent reading. According to Cohen et al., a standard model of word reading proposes that visual information is initially processed by occipito-temporal areas contra-lateral to the stimulated hemi-field. Then it is transferred to the visual word form system (VWFA), a left temporal region devoted to the processing of letter strings. Using fMRI, they identified a highly significant activation in the left fusiform gyrus (Talairach coordinates: $x = -42$, $y = -57$, $z = -6$) that was strictly unilateral and remarkably stable across subjects [80]. Since their research also included comparisons of activation from the right and left visual hemi-fields, they concluded that the VWFA lies at the convergence of retinotopically organized visual pathways and contain visual neurons with receptive fields in both hemi-fields. They hypothesize that the VWFA may be homologous to inferotemporal areas in the monkey where cells with wide receptive fields, selectivity to high-level visual features, and size and position invariance have been found. If this is the case, it is possible that the human VWFA holds a distributed representation of the visual shapes of letters such that specific alphabetic strings are distinguished and is thought to supply instantaneous recognition of learned letters, letter patterns, and unique words.

Van der Mark et al. researched areas of the fusiform gyrus for activations related to visual processing. Initially, they found a posterior–anterior measure of change to print specificity with higher anterior response to letter strings but higher posterior response to false-fonts. Additionally, there was a constant sensitivity to orthographic familiarity demonstrated by higher response for unfamiliar than familiar word-forms. These variations along the VWF-System could only be detected in controls. They used functional connectivity MRI (fcMRI) to correlate signal changes in a seed region with signal changes in other parts of the brain and reveal functional interactions between brain areas. Five non-overlapping seed regions of interest (ROIs; spheres with a 6 mm radius) centered on the VWFA of the fusiform gyrus and covering neighboring areas along a posterior–anterior axis in the left hemisphere were defined, with ROI3 being the VWFA itself. Results showed that functional connectivity in children with dyslexia was significantly reduced only between the VWFA proper (ROI3) and classical left hemispheric language related regions, including the inferior parietal lobule and the inferior frontal gyrus. Significantly greater connectivity for the dyslexia than the control group was observed between ROI3 and the left middle temporal and middle occipital gyrus, and between ROI4 and the left superior temporal gyrus and the left insula. The strength of the functional connections between VWFA (ROI3) and the left middle temporal gyrus and between ROI4 and the left superior temporal gyrus did not correlate significantly with the behavioral measures in either the control group or the children with dyslexia. Correlating these increases in connectivity does not reflect better performance, but instead compensation efforts. They conclude, as did Wolf, that dyslexics may not use the network in the same way as controls [81].

9. Evidence from diffusion tensor imaging

A "disconnection syndrome" in which functional connectivity of the relevant cortical networks in the left hemisphere is disrupted has been proposed as a potential basis for reading difficulties [82]. Diffusion Tensor Imaging (DTI), a technology similar to fMRI, allows probing the distance and direction of water molecule movement in the brain, producing form and orientation information about the underlying white matter structures [83]. White matter exhibits anisotropic water movement, with water molecules showing various degrees of diffusion in each direction. In typical DTI studies, diffusion images from at least six directions are analyzed using an ellipsoid tensor model—a symmetrical 3×3 matrix. Parallel and perpendicular diffusivities are then calculated and used to estimate properties of underlying tissues [84]. DTI has demonstrated a correlation between the microstructural integrity of the left temporo-parietal white matter and reading ability in dyslexic and control adults [85]. It seems that this technology could be instrumental in measuring not only the degree of connectedness between crucial brain features, but also in determining the amount of pressure needed by these systems to change functioning.

Fractional anisotropy (FA) is a related technology that is used to index structural information regarding a brain area. It measures the anisotropy of the diffusion of water molecules [86] and is sensitive to axonal density, size, myelination, and the coherence of organization of fibers within a voxel, thus providing an index of the structural integrity of white matter. FA is measured from 0 (isotropic diffusion) to 1 (anisotropic diffusion) [83]. Beaulieu et al. propose that FA may be reduced in poor readers due to a number of possible differences in the microstructural properties of white matter. These possible differences include reduced myelination, reduced axonal packing density, decreased axonal diameter, or reduced coherence of the orientation of axons within the region, all of which might impact the efficiency of communication (bandwidth) among cortical areas [87]. Further, their findings suggest that there are regional brain structural correlations over a wide range of reading ability even within a so-called normal population. Keller and Just examined the diffusivity in directions that are perpendicular to the principal axis of diffusion in anisotropic regions of white matter (radial diffusivity) or parallel to it (axial diffusivity). They suggest that the pattern of diffusivity effects signifies that the difference in FA between poor and good readers before remediation is due to initially higher radial diffusivity in the poor readers. Further indicating that the change in FA results from an alteration in some microstructural feature-myelination, packing density, or axon diameter- that affects radial diffusivity. By default, myelination is deemed the plausible mechanism of the microstructural change [88]. It is possible that extended, pressured practice affects the myelinated cortical thickness in key regions of the neuroanatomical correlates of the dual route reading model.

In a meta-analysis focusing on the foci of brain activity in a set of studies, Richlan, Kronbichler, and Wimmer used Activation Likelihood Estimation (ALE) to analyze for agreement by modeling each reported focus as the center of a Gaussian probability distribution. These distributions are then joined to create a whole-brain statistical map that estimates the likelihood of activation for each voxel. The data from 17 studies (12 fMRI and 5 PET) with a total number of 595 participants (294 dyslexics and 301 controls) were included. This approach resulted in three ALE maps: one, presenting brain regions with under-activation in dyslexic readers, another, presenting regions with over-activation and, finally, a subtraction map which allows a formal assessment of differences between the two maps. The results extracted 128 foci of reliable group differences (69 for dyslexic under-activation and 59 for dyslexic over-activation), and localized 80 input foci in the left hemisphere and only 48 in the right hemisphere. They found that 58% of the left and 48% of the right hemisphere foci were under-activation foci. The majority of activation abnormalities identified by separate maps were still present in the conservative thresholded difference map: under-activation in a large cluster in the left hemisphere reaching from dorsal inferior parietal to ventral occipito-temporal regions and to the middle temporal and the inferior frontal under-activation, with over-activation in left hemisphere anterior insula, primary motor cortex, lingual gyrus, caudate nuclei, thalamus and right hemisphere medial frontal cortex. These results provide support for a dysfunction of the VWFA engaged in visual-orthographic word recognition and a dysfunction of the left fusiform region affecting the build-up or the use of an orthographic word lexicon in recognition. Further, over-activation of the left lingual gyrus may reflect prolonged visual processing when dyslexic readers are confronted with a reading task [89].

Voxel Based Analysis (VBA) uses brain images normalized to a standard brain atlas and smoothed, before computing and comparing DTI properties for each individual voxel. This approach greatly reduces the typical biases of ROI analyses, though since it is typically less theoretically driven more drastic corrections for multiple comparisons are often required [90]. Moreau, Stonyer, McKay, and Waldie observed that many DTI studies have investigated significant differences in FA between dyslexic and typical readers, as well as identifying regions where FA values significantly correlate with performance on reading tasks, with problems in replication and little convergence of data. Using a very stringent process of examination, they identified research that used VBA to identify cortical coordinates where significant differences in FA existed between dyslexic and typical readers, and research that used VBA to locate cortical coordinates where FA significantly correlated with reading ability or performance on a reading-based task. Their results were extraordinary. The analysis of 47 foci from 5 experiments (99 subjects), where FA was significantly greater in typical compared to dyslexic readers, and the analysis of 17 foci from 2 experiments (52 subjects), where FA was significantly greater in dyslexic compared to typical readers, yielded no significant clusters when using FDR correction of 0.05. Further, the analysis of 42 foci from 9 experiments (500 subjects), where reading ability was significantly positively correlated with FA, and the analysis of 2 foci from 2 experiments (40 subjects), where reading ability was significantly negatively correlated with FA, also yielded no significant clusters when using FDR correction of 0.05. Studies of children and adults were analyzed separately. No significant clusters were produced when typical readers had significantly higher FA than dyslexic readers or when dyslexic readers had significantly greater FA than typical readers, regardless of age [90]. The fact that these results showed no systematic differences in fractional anisotropy between dyslexic and typical readers, or as a function of reading ability, after correcting for multiple comparisons, underscores the ambiguity inherent in brain research in spite of, or perhaps because of, cutting edge technologies. Hoppenbrouwers, Vandermosten, and Boets noted that despite appearing consistent, each one of the studies they included in their meta-analysis produced coordinates at different locations within the temporo-parietal region and corpus callosum [91]. In fact many studies have also reported differences and correlations in a range of other regions distributed widely throughout the cortex [59, 92]. Turkeltaub et al. pointed out that the software commonly used for these kinds of analysis, GingerALE 2.0.4, has since been updated too correct initial errors which made ALE analysis to lenient, therefore inadequately controlling for spurious findings [93].

10. Conclusion

There is little doubt that neurobiological investigation into the brain activations of struggling readers is messy and incomplete and fraught with misinformation. Reviews of international studies reveal many areas of agreement regarding the factors that result in dyslexia, but the characteristics of different languages and their orthographies introduce differences in the required processing skills. This is also seen in the unequal application of the Psycholinguistic Grain Size Theory, where transparent languages with a regular orthography are less affected than those opaque languages with many irregular words and derivatives. The contribution of RAN to understanding the neurobiological features of dyslexia appears to have global implications as this naming speed deficit has been found to be more common than even the phonological deficit in both regular and irregular orthographies. These methods and techniques used to investigate the manifestations of dyslexia worldwide have advanced the discussion in many useful ways.

Phonological processing and speed have long been in the forefront of international dyslexia research. Particularly in transparent orthographies, phonological impairments have supported the idea of lexical and sub-lexical routes of decoding that utilize different areas in the brain. Difficulties with phoneme blending often precede and contribute to a slower rate of reading. These processing weaknesses eventually produce students who display the dreaded Double Deficit- a condition that in many languages has been identified as the most severely incapacitating. However, in some languages, RAN is useful as a predictor of reading accuracy only in the early grades. Receptive vocabulary, often an important factor in less consistent orthographies, has been found to play a role in reading accuracy in more regular orthographies as readers become more experienced, but this seems to rely on specific language features that promote decoding based on lexical aspects of known, related words. So in languages where these language-specific patterns are prevalent, most dyslexics achieve high levels of reading accuracy but remain deficit in reading speed.

Research into the visual processing of struggling readers has focused mainly on the functions of the occipito-temporal reading circuit. Dysfunction in a variety of visuo-attentional skills such as visual search, visual recognition, and visual information processing has been documented in several languages, with both transparent and opaque orthographies. Interesting work in languages that use diacritical vowel markings which are absent after instruction emphasizes the theory that when grapheme-phoneme processing skills are weak, students are unable to develop strong connections in the orthographic lexicon to support further autonomous word recognition. In this case, the results also highlight the importance of visual accuracy and memory for the missing vowel markings. Generally, however, functional imaging studies reveal reduced reading related activation in a left ventral occipito-temporal brain area, often associated as an interface between visual orthographic codes and phonology and meaning. There is some assurance of parity for even complex visual languages like Urdu that RAN continues to be a reliable predictor of reading accuracy. Regardless, the question of effective interventions remains largely unanswered.

American researchers have addressed the problems inherent in dyslexia through new conceptualizations of fluency and definitions that acknowledge the crucial role played by the automatization of underlying subskills at the letter, letter-pattern, and word levels. They challenged the validity of the commonly held discrepancy definition of dyslexia which mandates that a student with reading difficulties can be labeled "dyslexic" only if they have an average or higher IQ. Research showed that there were no reliable differences in the brain functioning of poor readers with high IQs and poor readers with low IQs. The effects of instructional intervention have also been explored in studies with American students. Most of this research focuses on explicit instruction in the alphabetic principle and phonological processing. These efforts generally resulted in increases in the activation of left posterior superior temporal gyrus (STG), although processing speed remained unaffected. However, a novel study using visual hemisphere-specific stimulation has shown some advancement in the speed of processing of dyslexic readers. Matching struggling readers to either a left or right hemisphere intervention program by specific oral reading behaviors appears to be helpful in applying an effective remediation program. The differences in the composition of the intervention programs (the left hemisphere lessons are all phonologically decodable words and the right hemisphere lessons are all phonologically decodable non-words) apparently interact with the weak brain processing systems efficiently. The forced pressure of faster and faster recall appears to strengthen the pathways resulting in automatized recall. Brain activations of subjects who achieved levels of automatic processing (recall within 100–250 ms) revealed expected changes: pre-intervention, there was a great deal of diffuse activation in the frontal areas and in the right hemisphere, and post-intervention activation was much more focused bilaterally around the STG and postcentral gyrus with very little activation in the VWFA. Further these documented processing changes were discovered to directly support increases in reading speed in those students reaching automatic levels of visual processing. So, visual hemisphere-specific stimulation has emerged as an intervention tool that influences access to the VWFA in American dyslexic readers.

Other technologies also shed light on the functional connectivity of brain regions important to fluent reading, but, as always, must be scrutinized for reliability. It is well established that diffusion tensor imaging (DTI) and fractional anisotropy are useful tools for understanding the structural integrity of white matter. Many studies have investigated relationships between differences in FA and various reading abilities, and differences in FA in dyslexic and normal readers. Generally these studies identify left hemisphere under-activation from dorsal inferior parietal to ventral occipito-temporal regions and to the middle temporal and the inferior frontal under-activation, with over-activation in left hemisphere anterior insula, primary motor cortex, lingual gyrus, caudate nuclei, thalamus, and right hemisphere medial frontal cortex. However, many researchers have also commented that in spite of apparent consistency, there is substantial disparity in the coordinates locating specific activations in the temporo-parietal region and corpus callosum. These observations led to a careful, but controversial meta-analysis using voxel-based analysis (VBA) to identify cortical coordinates where significant differences in FA existed. These analyses found no systematic differences in FA between dyslexic and typical readers, or as a function of reading ability, and highlighted possible weaknesses in older versions of the software commonly used to make DTI analyses. Clearly, one must engage in this kind of research and rely on these results cautiously.

For many years, the only neurobiological research was done in adults, which did not allow investigation of the developing brain. Granted, it is very challenging to obtain reliable fMRI results with children, but new techniques and a more permissive environment are encouraging, and the promise of bringing new understandings to fruition as effective intervention practices continues to beckon. Instructional intervention that is designed to improve time-sensitive procedural rather than time-free declarative knowledge of grapheme-phoneme correspondences may overcome the temporal deficit in children by decreasing the over-connectivity of brain regions in the executive panel of working memory- that is the left and right inferior frontal gyrus, and increasing the connectivity between the left inferior frontal gyrus and the middle frontal gyrus (working memory) [94]. From a clinical or educational perspective, remediation seems most targeted and effective when it addresses an isolated disability [71]. The challenge in developing strong intervention tools is to make them engaging, accessible, and fun.

Saine et al. conducted a longitudinal intervention study designed to build a model of predictive values of reading fluency using three different instructional techniques to identify the most effective type of intervention for children with different profiles of core pre-reading skills. Their results show that a computerized remedial reading intervention called GraphoGame was the most successful in remediating reading fluency in Finnish children (7 years old) with deficits in letter knowledge, phonological awareness, and rapid automatized naming [95]. Perhaps reflecting its extremely shallow orthography, (there is full symmetric consistency between graphemes and phonemes and the simplest syllabic structure in the Finnish language) and the fairly long duration of intervention (66 hours), increases in fluency were found in both of the other treatments (remedial reading instruction and mainstream instruction) as well, with the least amount of growth shown in the mainstream group. However, evaluation of data by pre-reading profiles shows that all of the tested profile-types responded most strongly in the computerized reading program.

The GraphoGame program is similar to FlashWord in the structure of the phonological analysis, proceeding from early reading competencies to higher-level concepts, and in the forced, fast processing at the word-level. It was developed to affect the cognitive operations that constitute word reading: the visual identification of orthographic units, their transformation into an internal sound and articulation. This program's creators included the appearance of letters and words at an accelerating rate on the screen (although without hemisphere consideration) in an effort to improve automatized naming and visual recognition more effectively than flashcards [95]. The direct comparison of traditional instructional techniques to outcomes produced through a computer-based intervention underscores the power of these types of programs and their impact on the automatization of lexical and sub-lexical reading processes. Perhaps the power of technology in new applications will ultimately provide solutions for the long-suffering dyslexic readers, especially those of opaque orthographies.

Author details

Bobbie Jean Koen
University of Houston, Houston, Texas, United States

*Address all correspondence to: bjkoen@comcast.net

References

[1] Coltheart M, Curtis B, Atkins P, Haller M. Models of reading aloud: Dual route and parallel processing approaches. Psychological Review. 1993; **100**:589-608

[2] Shany M, Share DL. Subtypes of reading disability in a shallow orthography: A double dissociation between accuracy-disabled and rate-disabled readers of Hebrew. Annals of Dyslexia. 2011;**61**(1):64-84

[3] Coltheart M, Rastle K, Perry C, Langdon R, Ziegler J. DRC: A dual route cascaded model of visual word recognition and reading aloud. Psychological Review. 2001;**108**: 204-256

[4] Jiménez JE, Rodríguez C, Ramírez G. Spanish development in dyslexia: Prevalence, cognitive profile and home literacy experiences. Journal of Experimental Child Psychology. 2009; **103**:167-185

[5] Seymour PHK, Aro M, Erskine JM. Foundation literacy acquisition in European orthographies. British Journal of Psychology. 2003;**94**:143-174

[6] Hutzler F, Wimmer H. Eye movements of dyslexic children when reading in a regular orthography. Brain and Language. 2004;**89**:235-242

[7] Wolf M, Bowers PGP, Michael G. The double-deficit hypothesis for the developmental dyslexias. Journal of Educational Psychology. 1999;**91**(3): 415-438

[8] Galaburda AM, Rosen GD, Sherman GF. Individual variability in cortical organization: Its relationship to brain laterality and implications to function. Neuropsychologia. 1990;**28**(6):529-546

[9] Rezaie R, Panagiotis SG, Fletcher JM, Juranek J, Cirnio PT, Li Z, et al. The timing and strength of regional brain activation associated with word recognition in children with reading difficulties. Frontiers in Human Neuroscience. 2011;**5**:45

[10] Gross-Glenn K, Duara R, Barker WW, Loewenstein D, Chang JY, Yoshii F, et al. Positron emission tomographic studies during serial word-reading by normal and dyslexic adults. Journal of Clinical and Experimental Neuropsychology. 1991;**13**(4):531-544

[11] Filipek AP, Semrud-Clikeman JM, Steingard FR, Renshaw NP, Kennedy ND, Biederman NJ. Volumetric MRI analysis comparing subjects having attention-deficit hyperactivity disorder with normal controls. Neurology. 1997; **48**(3):589-601

[12] Constable RT, Ni W, Mencl E, Pugh K, Fulbright R, Shaywitz S, et al. Activation response to semantic and syntactic anomalies: An fMRI study. NeuroImage. 1998;**7**(4):S188-S188

[13] Layes S, Lalonde R, Rebai M. Reading speed and phonological awareness deficits among Arabic-speaking children with dyslexia. Dyslexia. 2015;**21**:81-95. DOI: 10.1002/dys.1491

[14] Wolf M. Proust and the Squid. New York: HarperCollins; 2007 295p

[15] Seymour PHK. Early reading development in European orthographies. In: Snowling MJ, Hulme C, editors. The Science of Reading: A Handbook. Oxford, England: Blackwell; 2005. pp. 296-315. DOI: 10.1002/9780470757642.ch16

[16] Landerl K, Ramus F, Moll K, Lyytinen H, Leppänen PH, Lohvansuu K, et al. Predictors of developmental dyslexia in European orthographies with varying complexity. Journal of Child

Psychology and Psychiatry. 2013;**54**(6): 686-694. DOI: 10.1111/jcpp.12029

[17] Ziegler JC, Goswami U. Reading acquisition, developmental dyslexia, and skilled reading across languages: A psycholinguistic grain size theory. Psychological Bulletin. 2005;**131**(1): 3-29. DOI: 10.1037/0033-2909.131.1.3

[18] Denckla MB, Rudel RG. Rapid 'automatized' naming (R.A.N.): Dyslexia differentiated from other learning disabilities. Neuropsychologia. 1976;**14**(4):471-479. DOI: 10.1016/ 0028-3932(76)90075-0

[19] Wolf M, Bowers PG, Biddle K. Naming-speed processes, timing, and reading: A conceptual review. Journal of Learning Disabilities. 2000;**33**(4):387-407. DOI: 10.1177/002221940003300409

[20] Wimmer H, Mayringer H, Landerl KP, Michael G. The double-deficit hypothesis and difficulties in learning to read a regular orthography. Journal of Educational Psychology. 2000;**92**(4):668-680. DOI: 10.1037/ 0022-O663.92.4.668

[21] Bowers P, Newby-Clark E. The role of naming speed within a model of reading acquisition. Reading and Writing. 2002;**15**(1):109-126

[22] Savage R, Frederickson N. Evidence of a highly specific relationship between rapid automatic naming of digits and text-reading speed. Brain and Language. 2005;**93**(2):152-159. DOI: 10.1016/ j.bandl.2004.09.005

[23] O'Brien BA, Wolf M, Lovett MW. A taxometric investigation of developmental dyslexia subtypes. Dyslexia. 2012;**18**(1):16-39. DOI: 10.1002/dys.1431

[24] Vaessen A, Blomert L. Long-term cognitive dynamics of fluent reading development. Journal of Experimental Child Psychology. 2010;**105**(3):213-231. DOI: 10.1016/j.jecp.2009.11.005

[25] Sprenger-Charolles L. Dyslexia subtypes in languages differing in orthographic transparency: English, French, and Spanish. Escritos de Psicología. 2011;**4**(2):5-16. DOI: 10.5231/ psy.writ.2011.17072

[26] Ziegler JC, Castel C, Pech-Georgel C, George F, Alario F-X, Perry C. Developmental dyslexia and the dual route model of reading: Simulating individual differences and subtypes. Cognition. 2008;**107**(1):151-178. DOI: 10.1016/j.cognition.2007.09.004

[27] Landerl K, Wimmer H, Frith U. The impact of orthographic consistency on dyslexia: A German-English comparison. Cognition. 1997;**63**(3): 315-334

[28] Mann V, Wimmer H. Phoneme awareness and pathways into literacy: A comparison of German and American children. Reading and Writing: An Interdisciplinary Journal. 2002;**15**(7-8): 653-682

[29] Landerl K, Wimmer H. Development of word reading fluency and spelling in a consistent orthography: An 8-year follow-up. Journal of Educational Psychology. 2008;**100**(1):150-161. DOI: 10.1037/ 0022-0663.100.1.150

[30] Thaler V, Ebner E, Wimmer H, Landerl K. Training reading fluency in dysfluent readers with high reading accuracy: Word specific effects but low transfer to untrained words. Annals of Dyslexia. 2004;**54**(1):89-113

[31] De Luca M, Borrelli M, Judica A, Spinelli D, Zoccolotti P. Reading words and pseudowords: An eye movement study of developmental dyslexia. Brain and Language. 2002;**80**(3):617-626. DOI: 10.1006/brln.2001.2637

[32] Wimmer H, Mayringer H, Landerl K. Poor reading: A deficit in skill-automatization or a phonological deficit? Scientific Studies of Reading. 1998;**2**(4):321-340. DOI: 10.1207/s1532799xssr0204_2

[33] Zoccolotti P, De Luca M, Di Pace E, Judica A, Orlandi M, Spinelli D. Markers of developmental surface dyslexia in a language (Italian) with high grapheme-phoneme correspondence. Applied PsychoLinguistics. 1999;**20**(2):191-216

[34] Zoccolotti P, De Luca M, Di Pace E, Gasperini F, Judica A, Spinelli D. Word length effect in early reading and in developmental dyslexia. Brain and Language. 2005;**93**(3):369-373. DOI: 10.1016/j.bandl.2004.10.010

[35] Tobia V, Marzocchi GM. Cognitive profiles of Italian children with developmental dyslexia. Reading Research Quarterly. 2014;**49**(4):437-452. DOI: 10.1002/rrq.77

[36] Park H-R, Uno A. Cognitive abilities underlying reading accuracy, fluency and spelling acquisition in Korean Hangul learners from grades 1 to 4: A cross-sectional study. Dyslexia. 2015;**21**(3):235-253. DOI: 10.1002/dys.1500

[37] Cho J-R, Mcbride-Chang C, Park S-G. Phonological awareness and morphological awareness: Differential associations to regular and irregular word recognition in early Korean Hangul readers. Reading and Writing: An Interdisciplinary Journal. 2008;**21**(3):255-274. DOI: DOI 10.1007/s11145-007-9072-z

[38] Ziegler JC, Bertrand D, Tóth D, Csépe V, Reis A, Faísca L, et al. Orthographic depth and its impact on universal predictors of reading: A cross-language investigation. Psychological Science. 2010;**21**(4):551-559. DOI: 10.1177/0956797610363406

[39] Georgiou GK, Parrila R, Papadopoulos TC, Harris KR. Predictors of word decoding and reading fluency across languages varying in orthographic consistency. Journal of Educational Psychology. 2008;**100**(3):566-580. DOI: 10.1037/0022-0663.100.3.566

[40] Wimmer H. Characteristics of developmental dyslexia in a regular writing system. Applied PsychoLinguistics. 1993;**14**(1):1-33

[41] Yap R, Van der Leij A. Word processing in dyslexics: An automatic decoding deficit? Reading and Writing: An Interdisciplinary Journal. 1993;**5**(3):261-279

[42] Bjaalid I-K, Hoien T, Lundberg I, Bjaalid I-K. The contribution of orthographic and phonological processes to word reading in young Norwegian readers. Reading and Writing. 1996;**8**(2):189-198

[43] Porpodas CD. Patterns of phonological and memory processing in beginning readers and spellers of Greek. Journal of Learning Disabilities. 1999;**32**(5):406-416. DOI: 10.1177/002221949903200506

[44] Puolakanaho A, Ahonen T, Aro M, Eklund K, Leppanen PHT, Poikkeus A-M, et al. Very early phonological and language skills: Estimating individual risk of reading disability. Journal of Child Psychology and Psychiatry. 2007;**48**(9):923-931. DOI: 10.1111/j.1469-7610.2007.01763.x

[45] Csépe V, Honbolygó F, Paavo HT, Leppänen PHT. The neural prerequisites of reading. International Journal of Psychophysiology. 2012;**85**(3):321-321. DOI: 10.1016/j.ijpsycho.2012.06.087

[46] Breznitz Z. Enhancing the reading of dyslexic children by reading acceleration and auditory masking.

Journal of Educational Psychology. 1997; **89**(1):103-113

[47] Frost R. Phonetic recoding of print and its effect on the detection of concurrent speech in amplitude-modulated noise. Cognition. 1991;**39**(3): 195-214. DOI: 10.1016/0010-0277(91) 90053-7

[48] Aro M, Wimmer H. Learning to read: English in comparison to six more regular orthographies. Applied PsychoLinguistics. 2003;**24**(4):621-635. DOI: 10.1017/S0142716403000316

[49] Talcott JB, Gram A, van Ingelghem M, Witton C, Stein JF, Toennessen FE. Impaired sensitivity to dynamic stimuli in poor readers of a regular orthography. Brain and Language. 2003;**87**(2): 259-266. DOI: 10.1016/S0093-934X(03) 00105-6

[50] Salmelin R, Helenius P. Functional neuroanatomy of impaired reading in dyslexia. Scientific Studies of Reading. 2004;**8**(3):257-272. DOI: 10.1207/ s1532799xssr0803_5

[51] Paulesu E, Demonet J-F, Fazio F, Mccrory E, Chanoine V, Brunswick N, et al. Dyslexia: Cultural diversity and biological unity. Science. 2001; **291**(5511):2165-2167. DOI: search. proquest.com.ezproxy.lib.uh.edu/ docview/743189855?accountid=7107

[52] Eden GF, Vanmeter JW, Rumsey JM, Maisog JM, Woods RP, Zeffiro TA. Abnormal processing of visual motion in dyslexia revealed by functional brain imaging. Nature. 1996;**382**(6586):66

[53] Vidyasagar TR, Pammer K. Dyslexia: A deficit in visuo-spatial attention, not in phonological processing. Trends in Cognitive Sciences. 2010;**14**(2):57-63. DOI: 10.1016/j.tics.2009.12.003

[54] Geiger G, Cattaneo C, Galli R, Pozzoli U, Lorusso ML, Facoetti A, et al. Wide and diffuse perceptual modes characterize dyslexics in vision and audition. Perception. 2008;**37**(11): 1745-1764. DOI: 10.1068/p6036

[55] Slaghuis W, Lovegrove W. The effect of field size and luminance on spatial-frequency-dependent visible persistence and specific reading disability. Bulletin of the Psychonomic Society. 1987;**25**(1):38-40

[56] Kim J, Davis C, Burnham D, Luksaneeyanawin S. The effect of script on poor readers' sensitivity to dynamic visual stimuli. Brain and Language. 2004;**91**(3):326-335. DOI: 10.1016/j. bandl.2004.05.001

[57] Schiff R, Katzir T, Shoshan N. Reading accuracy and speed of vowelized and unvowelized scripts among dyslexic readers of Hebrew: The road not taken. Annals of Dyslexia. 2013;**63**(2):171-185. DOI: 10.1007/ s11881-012-0078-0

[58] Geschwind N. Disconnexion syndromes in animals and man: Part I. 1965. Neuropsychology Review. 2010; **20**(2):128-157. DOI: 10.1007/ s11065-010-9131-0

[59] Deutsch GK, Dougherty RF, Bammer R, Siok WT, Gabrieli JDE, Wandell B. Children's reading performance is correlated with white matter structure measured by diffusion tensor imaging. Cortex. 2005;**41**(3): 354-363. DOI: 10.1016/S0010-9452(08) 70272-7

[60] Kronbichler M, Hutzler F, Staffen W, Mair A, Ladurner G, Wimmer H. Evidence for a dysfunction of left posterior reading areas in German dyslexic readers. Neuropsychologia. 2006;**44**(10):1822-1832. DOI: 10.1016/j. neuropsychologia.2006.03.010

[61] Farukh A, Vulchanova M. Predictors of reading in Urdu: Does deep orthography have an impact?

Dyslexia. 2014;**20**(2):146-166. DOI: 10.1002/dys.1474

[62] Goswami U. Reading, dyslexia and the brain. Educational Research. 2008; **50**(2):135-148. DOI: 10.1080/ 00131880802082625

[63] Attneave FBM, Hebb DO. The organization of behavior: A neuropsychological theory. The American Journal of Psychology. 1950; **63**(4):633. DOI: 10.2307/1418888

[64] Laberge D, Samuels SJ. Toward a theory of automatic information processing in reading. Cognitive Psychology. 1974;**6**(2):293-323. DOI: 10.1016/0010-0285(74)90015-2

[65] Kame'enui EJ, Simmons DC, Good RH, Harn BA. The use of fluency-based measures in early identification and evaluation of intervention efficacy in schools. In: Wolf M, editor. Dyslexia, Fluency, and the Brain. Parkton, MD: York Press; 2000. pp. 307-332

[66] Wolf M, Katzir-Cohen T. Reading Fluency and Its Intervention. Scientific Studies of Reading. 2001;**5**(3):211-239. DOI: 10.1207/S1532799XSSR0503_2

[67] Kame'enui EJ. A new paradigm; Responsiveness to intervention. Teaching Exceptional Children. 2007; **39**(5):6-7

[68] Frith U. Brain, mind and behavior in dyslexia. In: Hulme C, Snowling M, editors. Dyslexia: Biology, Cognition and Intervention. London, England: Whurr; 1997. pp. 1-19

[69] Stuebing KK, Fletcher JM, Ledoux JM, Lyon GR, Shaywitz SE, Shaywitz BA. Validity of IQ-discrepancy classifications of reading disabilities: A meta-analysis. American Educational Research Journal. 2002;**39**(2):469-518

[70] Machek GR, Nelson JM. School psychologists' perceptions regarding the practice of identifying reading disabilities: Cognitive assessment and response to intervention considerations. Psychology in the Schools. 2010;**47**(3): 230-245. DOI: 10.1002/pits.20467

[71] Tanaka H, Black JM, Hulme C, Stanley LM, Kesler SR, Whitfield-Gabrieli S, et al. The brain basis of the phonological deficit in dyslexia is independent of IQ. Psychological Science. 2011;**22**(11):1442-1451. DOI: 10.1.177/095679761.141.952.1

[72] Katzir T, Kim Y, Wolf M, Kennedy B, Lovett M, Morris R. The relationship of spelling recognition, ran, and phonological awareness to reading skills in older poor readers and younger reading-matched controls. Reading and Writing: An Interdisciplinary Journal. 2006;**19**(8):845-872. DOI: 10.1007/ s11145-006-9013-2

[73] Shaywitz B, Shaywitz S, Blachman B, Pugh K, Fulbright R, Skudlarski P, et al. Development of left occipitotemporal systems for skilled reading in children after a phonologically-based intervention. Biological Psychiatry. 2004;**55**(9): 926-934. DOI: 10.1016/j.biopsych. 2003.12.019

[74] Simos PG, Breier JI, Fletcher JM, Bergman E, Papanicolaou AC. Cerebral mechanisms involved in word reading in dyslexic children: A magnetic source imaging approach. Cerebral Cortex. 2000;**10**(8):809-816

[75] Bakker DJ, Vinke J. Effects of hemisphere-specific stimulation on brain activity and reading in dyslexics. Journal of Clinical and Experimental Neuropsychology. 1985;**7**(5):505-525. DOI: 10.1080/01688638508401282

[76] Lorusso M, Facoetti A, Paganoni P, Pezzani M, Molteni M. Effects of visual hemispheric specific stimulation versus reading – focused training in dyslexic children. Neuropyschological

Rehabilitation. 2006;**16**(2):194-212. DOI: 10.1080/09602010500145620

[77] Masutto C, Fabbro F. FlashWord: Training neuropsicologico per la dislessia. Italy: Editrice TecnoScuola, Gorizia (GO); 1995

[78] Koen BJ, Hawkins J, Zhu X, Jansen B, Fan W, Johnson S, et al. The location and effects of visual hemisphere-specific stimulation on reading fluency in children with the characteristics of dyslexia. Journal of Learning Disabilities. 2018;**51**(4):399-415. DOI: 10.1177/0022219417711223

[79] Shaywitz BA, Shaywitz SE, Pugh KR, Mencl WE, Fulbright RK, Skudlarski P, et al. Disruption of posterior brain systems for reading in children with developmental dyslexia. Biological Psychiatry. 2002;**52**(2): 101-110. DOI: 10.1016/S0006-3223(02) 01365-3

[80] Cohen L, Dehaene S, Naccache L, Lehricy S, Dehaene-Lambertz G, Hnaff M-A, et al. The visual word form area. Brain. 2000;**123**(2):291-307

[81] van Der Mark S, Klaver P, Bucher K, Maurer U, Schulz E, Brem S, et al. The left occipitotemporal system in reading: Disruption of focal fMRI connectivity to left inferior frontal and inferior parietal language areas in children with dyslexia. NeuroImage. 2011;**54**(3): 2426-2436. DOI: 10.1016/j.neuroimage. 2010.10.002

[82] Horwitz B, Jeffries KJ, Braun AR. Functional connectivity among language areas during speech production. NeuroImage. 2000;**11**(5): S284-S284

[83] Assaf Y, Pasternak O. Diffusion tensor imaging (DTI)-based white matter mapping in brain research: A Review. Journal of Molecular Neuroscience. 2008;**34**(1):51-61. DOI: 10.1007/s12031-007-0029-0

[84] Moreau D, Stonyer JE, McKay NS, Waldie KE. No evidence for systematic white matter correlates of dyslexia: An activation likelihood estimation meta-analysis. Brain Research. 2018;**1683**: 36-47. DOI: 10.1016/j.brainres. 2018.01.014

[85] Klingberg T, Hedehus M, Temple E, Salz T, Gabrieli JDE, Moseley ME, et al. Microstructure of temporo-parietal white matter as a basis for reading ability: Evidence from diffusion tensor magnetic resonance imaging. Neuron. 2000;**25**(2):493-500. DOI: 10.1016/ S0896-6273(00)80911-3

[86] Basser PJ, Pierpaoli C. Microstructural and physiological features of tissues elucidated by quantitative-diffusion-tensor MRI. Journal of Magnetic Resonance. 2011;**213**(2):560-570. DOI: 10.1016/j.jmr.2011.09.022

[87] Beaulieu C, Plewes C, Paulson LA, Roy D, Snook L, Concha L, et al. Imaging brain connectivity in children with diverse reading ability. NeuroImage. 2005;**25**(4):1266-1271. DOI: 10.1016/j.neuroimage.2004.12.053

[88] Keller TA, Just MA. Altering cortical connectivity: Remediation-induced changes in the white matter of poor readers. Neuron. 2009;**64**(5):624-631. DOI: 10.1016/j.neuron.2009.10.018

[89] Richlan F, Kronbichler M, Wimmer H. Functional abnormalities in the dyslexic brain: A quantitative meta-analysis of neuroimaging studies. Human Brain Mapping. 2009;**30**: 3299-3308. DOI: 10.1002/hbm.20752

[90] Soares JM, Magalhães R, Moreira PS, Sousa A, Ganz E, Sampaio A, et al. A hitchhiker's guide to functional magnetic resonance imaging. Frontiers in Neuroscience. 2016;**10**:515. DOI: 10.3389/fnins.2016.00515

[91] Hoppenbrouwers M, Vandermosten M, Boets B. Autism as a disconnection

syndrome: A qualitative and quantitative review of diffusion tensor imaging studies. Research in Autism Spectrum Disorders. 2014;**8**(4):387-412. DOI: 10.1016/j.rasd.2013.12.018

[92] Rimrodt SL, Peterson DJ, Denckla MB, Kaufmann WE, Cutting LE. White matter microstructural differences linked to left perisylvian language network in children with dyslexia. Cortex. 2010;**46**(6):739-749. DOI: 10.1016/j.cortex.2009.07.008

[93] Turkeltaub PE, Eickhoff SB, Laird AR, Fox M, Wiener M, Fox P. Minimizing within-experiment and within-group effects in activation likelihood estimation meta-analyses. Human Brain Mapping. 2012;**33**(1):1-13. DOI: 10.1002/hbm.21186

[94] Richards TL, Berninger VW. Abnormal fMRI connectivity in children with dyslexia during a phoneme task: Before but not after treatment. Journal of Neurolinguistics. 2008;**21**(4): 294-304. DOI: 10.1016/j.jneuroling. 2007.07.002

[95] Saine NL, Lerkkanen M-K, Ahonen T, Tolvanen A, Lyytinen H. Predicting word-level reading fluency outcomes in three contrastive groups: Remedial and computer-assisted remedial reading intervention, and mainstream instruction. Learning and Individual Differences. 2010;**20**:402-414. DOI: 10.1016/j.lindif.2010.06.004

Section 5

Early Intervention

Chapter 7

INA Early Intervention for Babies at Risk

Hagit Friedman, Marina Soloveichick, Amir Kushnir, Chava Kasher, Caroline Barmatz and Omer Bar-Yosef

Abstract

Brain and nervous system development are experience dependent. Indeed, the sequence of development is laid out genetically, but early environmental events are major contributors to the system's development and optimal functioning. Various fetal injuries and birth trauma make babies vulnerable to developmental problems: cerebral palsy, seizures, abnormal muscle tone, delayed developmental milestones, sensory integration, and more. Our goal in the study presented here was to improve the neurodevelopmental track of babies at risk using Infant Neural Aquatic. Parent and baby dyads who met initial criteria were recruited for a 5–6 months intervention period through an open invitation, followed by a conversation and signing informed consent. In the beginning and end of intervention period, participants completed questionnaires, and developmental features of the babies were assessed using analysis of neuro-motor and vocal characteristics. Significant neurodevelopmental delta between values at the end and beginning of intervention period, comparing intervention and control, is described, and the strength of INA specific intervention tool is analyzed.

Keywords: brain development, brain injury, early neurodevelopment, early intervention, developmental time windows, developmental insult, premature babies

1. Introduction

1.1 Early intervention

In the old Talmud, an imbecile, deaf-mute, and a minor were included in the same category related to religious obligations (Baba Kama 55 page B). This approach was explained as probably the earliest expression of the significance and power of early intervention—for babies and for disabled people.

In recent decades, we return to this approach and look for suitable and efficient early intervention models in order to successfully cope with developmental insults.

Training with babies in an aquatic setting has been found to benefit and promote infant health and development [1–3], being based on the physical properties of water and their physiological outcomes on the neuromotor [4–6], cardiovascular [7, 8], and respiratory functions [3]. Specifically, training with babies in an aquatic setting adapted for young babies with developmental risk may strengthen the function of autonomic parasympathetic nervous system and improve the development of neural circuits through better brain perfusion and sensory-motor training [1, 2, 9, 10].

In warm water, increased environmental pressure advances deep lung ventilation and higher lymphatic and venous return from the periphery; higher levels of blood and lymph entering the heart's right atrium cause slight bradycardia, producing a calming effect; most important for these infants, the water buoyant force causes the proprioceptors to cease registration of gravity; and an automatic reduction of muscle tone ensues. The benefits of reduced muscle tone linger for some hours following immersion. In these beneficial conditions, training is most effective both for sensory, emotional, and neuromotor purposes, and active parent role in this process is an additional advantage.

Training with young babies at risk, in an aquatic setting, may not cure severe brain lesions such as cerebral palsy; however, implying specific training approaches in specific developmental time windows may allow early effective intervention [11–15] which may eventually improve brain development.

This was our basic concept when we started our journey into the project, yet our findings showed us that our training protocol may have a deep neuro-power, more than we could foresee.

1.2 Early brain development and brain lesions

Neurodevelopmental syndromes are a continuously growing issue. These are impairments in the growth and development of the brain and CNS which appear in a variety of emotional, cognitive, motor, and social skills. One most important question when diagnosing and treating young children concerns the critical developmental time window through which chances for improvement would be strongest. Considering the fragility of young babies who are at developmental risk and the general tendency to postpone definite developmental diagnosis, the consideration of intervention should include neurological background of developmental mile stones.

During fetal development, a temporary assembly progresses in the subcortical future white matter, situated between the intermediate zone and the developing cortical plate, named cortical subplate [16]. As widely described in our recent paper [17], the subplate is thickest around the time of high production of oligodendrocyte father cells (29 weeks PMA), and is absorbed gradually until around 4 months post-term, with relocation of fiber terminals into the cortex [18, 19]. Most of its networks run through the (future) periventricular white matter. The size and duration of the subplate visibility correspond with cortical fiber complexity, being considered a recent phylogenetic structure that enables the increasing complexity of cortical circuitry [20].

The cortical subplate is a transmission complex for the neural projections of the developing cortical circuits and a regulating component that orchestrates neural network activity [21, 22]. Hence, subplate neurons are important for precise wiring and functionality of the cerebral cortex—they make initial temporary synapses between thalamic axons and their destinations in the early C4 layer [23].

SCP neurons, with their numerous synaptic contacts, are important factors that influence cortical development and ripening [24–26]. In the time gap of their presence, the SCP neural circuits are prone to hypoxic insult [27], which may cause long-term influence on brain development and functional deficits in various aspects. The time window of SCP circuits' high action is also the time window when young infants born premature make their first surviving out of utero.

1.3 Neurodevelopmental impairments

Neurodevelopmental impairments range from MND (minimal brain deficit) to ASD (autism spectrum disorder) and CP (cerebral palsy) [28–34]. Despite recent technological and scientific advance, there is currently no cure for severe neurodevelopmental impairments. However, various therapies may reduce the traumatic effect of brain lesions when diagnosed and treated during specific time windows in early infancy. Hence, the first weeks of baby's life may be critical for brain development through early and effective intervention.

The babies participating in our study were born premature and participated in this research during cortical subplate activity time window. Average birth percentage of preterm babies is around 10% and it is continuously rising. Prematurity is the global second frequent cause of death among babies. Although new medical tools enable more premature babies to live, many are at high risk for brain damage [29, 33, 35, 36] and neurodevelopmental insults [30, 34].

For example, cerebral palsy in premature neonates is caused mainly by developmental brain injury at the white matter of the brain—periventricular leucomalacia (PVL), due to bleeding in the brain (IVH, ICH), oxygen or blood deprivation (hypoxia, anoxia) in the brain [29, 32, 33]. Periventricular leucomalacia may cause severe, long-term damage to brain tissue [37–40]. Common symptoms of CP include lack of muscle coordination while performing voluntary movements (ataxia), and stiff or tight muscles and exaggerated reflexes (spasticity) with associated cognitive impairments.

Autism spectrum disorder (ASD) is the joint name for neurodevelopmental impairments characterized by abnormal social interaction, communication, limited range of activities and areas of interest [41], and typical motor impairments [42–53]. Being considered as sharing a similar mechanistic basis [54], previous ASD subcategories were unified under DSM5 (2013), and the classification today is based on severity of symptoms and level of disability.

There is a remarkable increase in the number of children diagnosed with ASD over the past 30 years, from less than 0.1% [55, 56] to ~1% [57] and more. Among infants at risk, premature infants have a five times higher risk of developing ASD, and a significantly high incidence of autistic symptoms was identified in premature infants [58, 59]. Changes in diagnostic criteria, different assessment tools, and increased public awareness may be only partially responsible for the increase in ASD epidemiology [60]. Studies indicate that genetic, neurological [59, 61–66], and environmental [67–72] factors are involved in the emergence of autism spectrum disorder (ASD).

Prenatal exposure to particulate matter solid fuels and traffic-related air pollutants, especially in the third trimester of prenatal development [67], link the ambient epigenetic aspects with internal genetic vulnerability due to lower, enzymatically based, removal ability of harmful remnants from infant's body. Indeed, these findings are in agreement with recent neurological understanding about the developmental time window of subcortical plate (SCP) during late prenatal and early postnatal period.

Early and effective intervention, through the important developmental time window of cortical subplate activity, may minimize neurological and functional deficits.

2. Basics of INA intervention approach

We have developed a unique training model for water—INA (Infant Neural Aquatics). The model consists of repetitive bilateral motor training and sustained moderate aerobic activity and their influence on desensitization and reprocessing of adverse events in utero and after birth.

After parents signed informed consent, INA was conducted in the hydrotherapy pool— babies were placed in warm water in vertical and horizontal positions, supported by the buoyancy of water and the caring hands of parent or therapist. Training started with a set of pre-structured movements through which parents practice handling of the infant in the water, in a way that enables free and integrated movement, eye contact, vocal communication, and increased confidence.

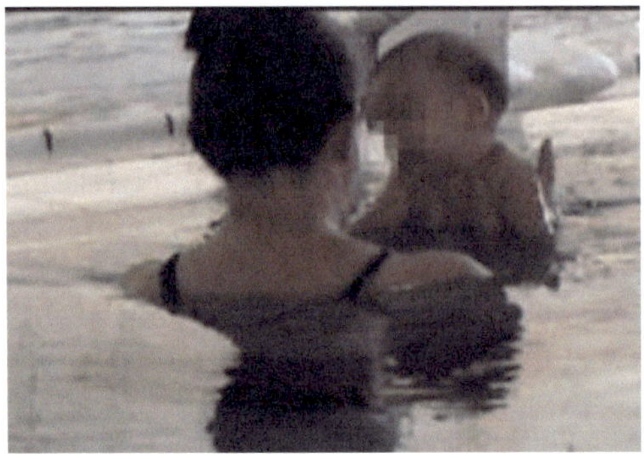

Figure 1.
INA (Infant Neural Aquatics) approach at work: Encouraging eye contact.

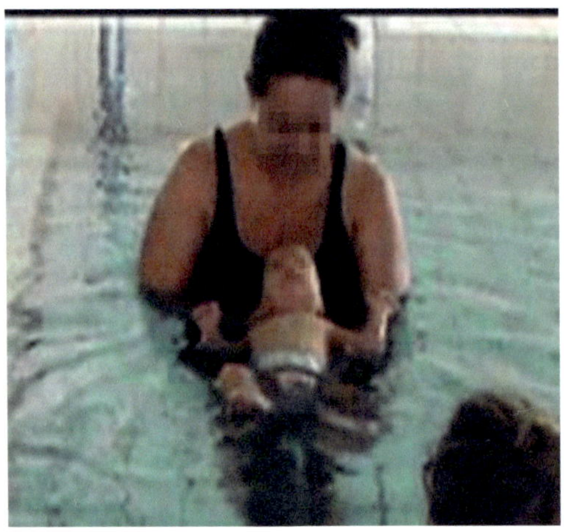

Figure 2.
INA (Infant Neural Aquatics) approach at work: Relaxed floating.

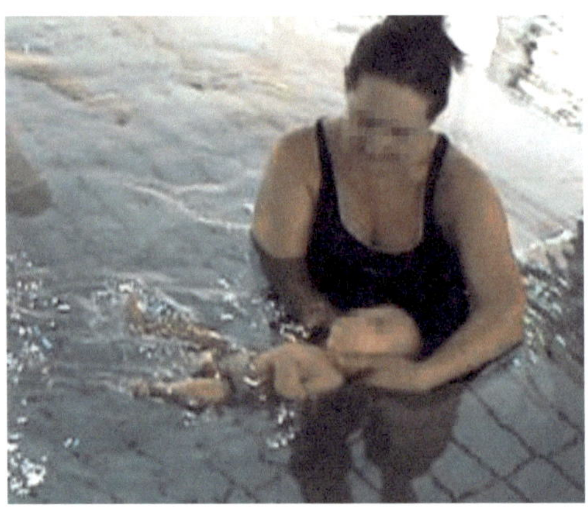

Figure 3.
INA (Infant Neural Aquatics) approach at work: 8 shape delicate mobilization.

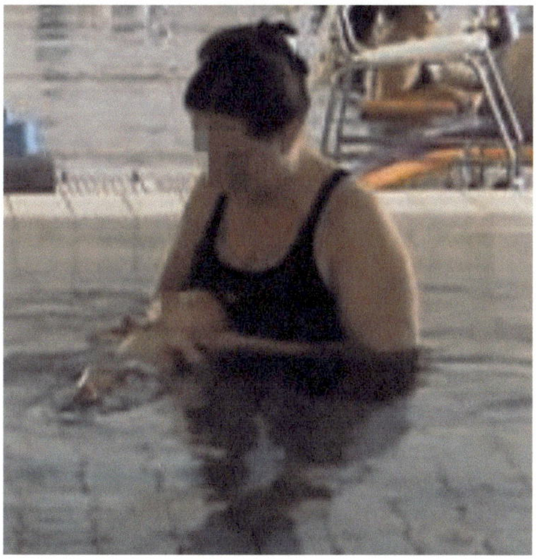

Figure 4.
INA (Infant Neural Aquatics) approach at work: Passive mobilizatio.

Working technique employed was modified for young and prematurely born Infants, including: passive mobilization, various rotations, relaxed floating, 8 shape delicate mobilization when the infant is supported under occiput and rib cage. Infants were video recorded during water sessions, under water and above water, once a week along 14 consecutive weeks (**Figures 1–4**).

3. Developmental track of babies

Developmental track of the babies with early intervention employing the INA approach was conducted at fixed time points using the non-intrusive General Movements (GM) tool [73–75]. The babies showed about 70% delta in developmental improvement comparing w/wo INA when the babies were around 55 wPMA.

Using the developmental tool ABAS (Adaptive Behavioral Assessment Scale) [76], the children showed about 40% delta in developmental improvement comparing w/wo INA, when the babies were around 1.5 years old (**Graphs 1, 2**).

Intervention group. 78.27% of the subjects got the same results in delta1 and delta2 (for 8.70% both delta are equal 0 and for 69.57% both delta were equal 1), 21.74% of the subjects did not get the same results in delta1 and delta2—delta1 = 1 and delta2 = 0 (no opposite cases). We calculated the kappa coefficient (system consistency) = 0.3575 (confidence limit 95% is −0.0242 till 0.7393). We conducted McNemar's Test (significance of results), P = 0.0625.

Control group. 87.50% of the subjects got the same results in delta1 and delta2 (for 66.67% both delta were equal 0 and for 20.83% both delta are equal 1), 12.50% of the subjects did not get the same results in delta1 and delta2—delta1 = 0 and delta2 = 1 (no opposite cases). We calculated kappa coefficient (system consistency) = 0.6897 (confidence limit 95% is 0.3774 till 1.000). We conducted McNemar's Test (significance of results), P = 0.2500.

In order to test if group (w/wo early intervention) and the babies' preliminary grades were dependent, we used Fisher Exact test and got non-significant result (P = 0.5806), which proves no link between group (w/wo early intervention) and babies' developmental grade. In order to test if group (intervention/control) and the babies' grades at 55 wPMA were dependent, we used Fisher Exact test and got

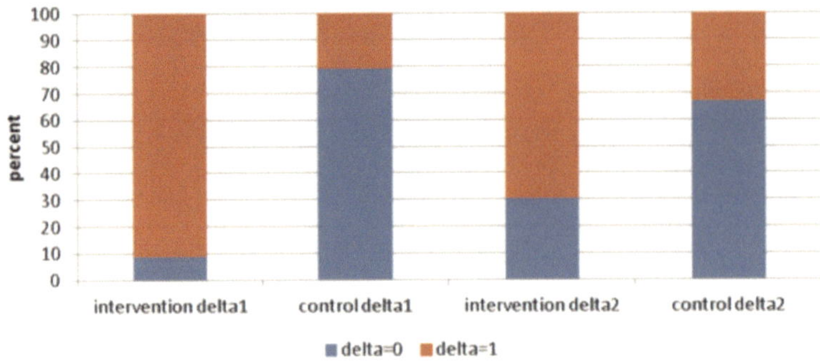

Graph 1.
Difference in developmental tracks between before and after early intervention period (delta), in group with INA (blue) compared to group without INA (red), at the age of 55 wPMA (delta1) and at the age of 1.5 years (delta2).

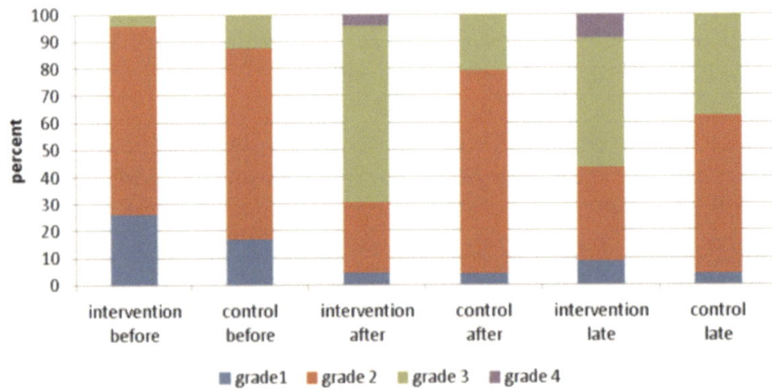

Graph 2.
Developmental grades before, immediately after, and 1 year after early intervention period.

significant result (P = 0.0016), which proves a link between intervention and infant early developmental grade.

In order to test if group's grade (intervention/control) and delta1 were dependent, we used Fisher Exact test and got significant result (P < 0.0001). In the intervention group. 8.70% got delta = 0, and in the control group. 79.17% got delta = 0. In order to test if group's grade (intervention/control) and delta2 were dependent, we used Fisher Exact test and got significant result (P = 0.0199). In the intervention group. 30.43% of delta = 0, and in the control group. 66.67% got delta = 0.

4. Conclusions, applicative potential, and future aims

Our results show significant improvement in developmental tracks of babies receiving INA compared to babies who did not, that is, delta in developmental tracks, between before and after early intervention, is ~40% higher when babies receive INA as observed without INA.

Screening of our videos, recording INA practice with the babies, we interpret that in addition to the significant benefits of the water's physical environment (described above), INA model functions as a therapeutic tool for the babies who experienced a trauma, much like the modern variants of EMDR (Eye Movement Desensitization and Reprocessing) model [77]. The bilateral passive and active stimulation and movement during INA training cause a scheduled activation of both right and left cortical hemispheres, unlock the traumatic experience in the right hemisphere, promote new connections in interhemispheric neural cycles, contributing to the high delta scores in the participants who received INA compared with those who did not.

We assume that longer intervention periods would keep the high delta scores to older age, allowing the brain more training and a longer period of enhanced conditions.

In the next stage of the project, we define the correlation between concentration curves of biomarkers related to brain injury in the participants' body fluids, and neuro-developmental track.

Indeed, the research described here directs the light on a certain vulnerable group of babies. However, the scientific and clinical products of this project, when properly tuned, may be successfully applied to various groups who are at developmental risk—children and youth diagnosed with post-trauma, or under extreme/acute emotional load, etc.

Acknowledgements

This scientific work is dedicated to my dear parents for their unlimited love and care.
We wish to thank:
The parents of the babies for their trust and cooperation.
The hydro therapists at Sheba MC Rehabilitation Pool for their collaboration.
The Haifa University Research Dean Fund for their generous support.
The Magi-Adelis Research Fund for their generous support.
The National Institute for Psychobiology in Israel, for their generous support.

Author details

Hagit Friedman[1*], Marina Soloveichick[2], Amir Kushnir[3], Chava Kasher[4], Caroline Barmatz[5] and Omer Bar-Yosef[6]

1 Faculty of Health Sciences, University of Haifa, Haifa, Israel

2 NICU, Carmel Medical Center, Haifa, Israel

3 NICU, Bar-Ilan University, Faculty of Medicine, Israel

4 NICU, Sheba Medical Center, Israel

5 Hydrotherapy, Sheba Medical Center, Israel

6 Pediatric Neurology, Safra Children's Hospital, Sheba Medical Center, Israel

*Address all correspondence to: drhagitfriedman@gmail.com

References

[1] Vignochi C. Effect of aquatic physical therapy on pain and state of sleep and wakefulness among stable preterm newborns in neonatal intensive care units. Revista Brasileira de Fisioterapia. 2011;**14**(3):214-220

[2] Zelazo PR, Weiss MJ. Infant swimming behaviors: Cognitive control and the influence of experience. Journal of Cognition and Development. 2006; 7(1):1-25

[3] Ahrendt L. The influence of infant swimming on the frequency of disease during the first year of life. In: Eriksson BE, Gullstrand L, editors. Proceedings of the XII FINA World Congress on Sports Medicine. Göteborg: Chalmers Reproservice; 1997. pp. 130-142

[4] Attermeier S. The use of water as a modality to treat an infant with mild neurological dysfunction. A case report. Physical & Occupational Therapy in Pediatrics. 1983;**3**(1):53-57

[5] Ahrendt L. The influence of water programs on infants' motor development. In: Kamp et al, editors. Advances in Motor Development and Learning in Infancy. Proceedings of the First World Congress on Motor Development and Learning in Infancy. Enschede: Print Partners Ipskamp;2001. pp. 85-88

[6] Getz M et al. Effects of aquatic interventions in children with neuromotor impairments: A systematic review of the literature. Clinical Rehabilitation. 2006a;**20**(11):927-937

[7] Goksor E et al. Bradycardic response during submersion in infant swimming. Acta Paediatrica. 2002;**91**(3):307-312

[8] Sweeney JK. Neonatal hydrotherapy: An adjunct to developmental intervention in an intensive care nursery setting. Physical & Occupational Therapy in Pediatrics. 1983;**3**(1):39-52

[9] Stein J. Motor development, the brain, and aquatic therapy. Aquatic Therapy Journal. 2004;**6**(2):19-23

[10] Wilcock D et al. Physiological response to water immersion: A method for sport recovery. Sports Medicine. 2006;**36**(9):747-766

[11] Nordhove SM et al. Early intervention improves behavioral outcomes for preterm infants: Randomized controlled trial. Pediatrics. 2012;**129**:e9

[12] Spittle AJ et al. Improving the outcome of infants born at <30 weeks' gestation – A randomized controlled trial of preventative care at home. BMC Pediatrics. 2009;**9**:73

[13] Orton J et al. Do early intervention programs improve cognitive and motor outcomes for preterm infants after discharge? A systematic review. Developmental Medicine and Child Neurology. 2009;**51**(11):851-859

[14] Guzzetta A et al. The effects of preterm infant massage on brain electrical activity. Developmental Medicine and Child Neurology. 2011

[15] Hernandez-Reif M et al. Preterm infants show reduced stress behaviors and activity after 5 days of massage therapy. Infant Behavior & Development. 2007;**30**:557-561

[16] Kostovic I, Rakic P. Developmental history of the transient subplate zone in the visual and somatosensory cortex of the macaque monkey and human brain. The Journal of Comparative Neurology. 1990;**297**:441-470

[17] Friedman H et al. Neuroplasticity in young age: Computer-based early

Neurodevelopment and Neurodevelopmental Disease neurodevelopment classifier. Ch. 3. In: Chaban V, editor. Neuroplasticity–Insights of Neural Organization. London, United Kingdom: IntechOpen; 2018

[18] Kostovic I, Judas M. Prolonged coexistence of transient and permanent circuitry elements in the developing cerebral cortex of fetuses and preterm infants. Developmental Medicine and Child Neurology. 2006;**48**:388-393

[19] Luhmann HJ, Kilb W, Hanganu-Opatz IL. Subplate cells: Amplifiers of neuronal activity in the developing cerebral cortex. Frontiers in Neuroanatomy. 2009;**3**(19):1-12

[20] Kanold PO, Luhmann HJ. The subplate and early cortical circuits. Annual Review of Neuroscience. 2010; **33**:23-48

[21] Voigt T, Opitz T, De Lima AD. Synchronous oscillatory activity in immature cortical network is driven by GABAergic preplate neurons. The Journal of Neuroscience. 2001;**21**(22): 8895-8905

[22] Yang JW, Hanganu-Opatz IL, Sun JJ, Luhmann HJ. Three patterns of oscillatory activity differentially synchronize developing neocortical networks in vivo. The Journal of Neuroscience. 2009;**29**:9011-9025

[23] Zhao C, Kao JP, Kanold PO. Functional excitatory microcircuits in neonatal cortex connect thalamus and layer 4. The Journal of Neuroscience. 2009;**29**(49):15479-15488

[24] Hirsch S, Luhmann HJ. Pathway-specificity in N-methyl-d-aspartate receptor-mediated synaptic inputs onto subplate neurons. Neuroscience. 2008; **153**:1092-1102

[25] Kanold PO, Kara P, Reid RC, Shatz CJ. Role of subplate neurons in functional maturation of visual cortical columns. Science. 2003;**301**:521-525

[26] Kanold PO, Shatz CJ. Subplate neurons regulate maturation of cortical inhibition and outcome of ocular dominance plasticity. Neuron. 2006;**51**: 627-638

[27] Perkins L, Hughes E, Srinivasan L, et al. Exploring cortical subplate evolution using MRI of the fetal brain. Developmental Neuroscience. 2008;**30**: 211-220

[28] Allen MC. Neurodevelopmental outcomes of preterm infants. Current Opinion in Neurology. 2008;**21**(2):123

[29] Bassan H et al. Neurodevelopmental outcome in survivors of periventricular hemorrhagic infarction. Pediatrics. 2007;**120**(4):785-792

[30] Kiechl-Kohlendorfer U et al. Adverse neurodevelopmental outcome in preterm infants: Risk factor profiles for different gestational ages. Acta Paediatrica. 2009;**98**(5):792-796

[31] Kinney HC. The near-term (late preterm) human brain and risk for periventricular leukomalacia: A review. Seminars in Perinatology. 2006;**30**(2): 81-88

[32] Roze E et al. Functional outcome at school age of preterm infants with periventricular hemorrhagic infarction. Pediatrics. 2009;**123**(6):1493-1500

[33] Volpe JJ. Brain injury in premature infants: A complex amalgam of destructive and developmental disturbances. Lancet Neurology. 2009; **8**(1):110-124

[34] Woodward LJ et al. Neonatal MRI to predict neurodevelopmental outcomes in preterm infants. The New England

Journal of Medicine. 2006;**355**(7): 685-694

[35] Han TR, Bang MS, Lim JY, Yoon BH, Kim IW. Risk factors of cerebral palsy in preterm infants. American Journal of Physical Medicine & Rehabilitation. 2002;**81**(4):297-303

[36] Volpe JJ. Cerebral White matter injury of the preterm infant-more common than you thinks (commentaries). Pediatrics. 2003;**112**: 176-180

[37] Larroque B, Ancel PY, Marret S, Marchand L, André M, Arnaud C, et al. EPIPAGE Study group. Neurodevelopmental disabilities and special care of 5-year-old children born before 33 weeks of gestation (the EPIPAGE study): A longitudinal cohort study. Lancet. 2008;**371**(9615): 813-820

[38] Smyser CD, Snyder AZ, Shimony JS, Mitra A, Inder TE, Neil JJ. Resting-state network complexity and magnitude are reduced in prematurely born infants. Cerebral Cortex. 2016; **26**(1):322-333

[39] Fischi-Gómez E, Vasung L, Meskaldji DE, Lazeyras F, Borradori-Tolsa C, Hagmann P, et al. Structural brain connectivity in school-age preterm infants provides evidence for impaired networks relevant for higher order cognitive skills and social cognition. Cerebral Cortex. 2014;**25**(9): 2793-2805

[40] Salmaso N, Jablonska B, Scafidi J, Vaccarino FM, Gallo V. Neurobiology of premature brain injury. Nature Neuroscience. 2014;**17**(3):341-346

[41] American Psychiatric Association. Diagnostic and Statistical Manual of Mental Disorders (DSM-IV). 4th ed. Washington, DC: American Psychiatric Association; 2000

[42] Kanner L. Autistic disturbances of affective contact. The Nervous Child. 1943;**2**:217-250

[43] Kanner L, Lesser LI. Early infantile autism. Pediatric Clinics of North America. 1958;**5**:711-730

[44] Asperger H. Die “Autistischen Psychopathen” im Kindesalter. Archiv für Psychiatrie und Nervenkrankheiten. 1944;**117**:132-135

[45] Damasio AR, Maurer RG. A neurological model for childhood autism. Archives of Neurology. 1978;**35**: 777-786

[46] Nebel MB, Joel SE, Muschelli J, Barber AD, Caffo BS, Pekar JJ, et al. Disruption of functional organization within the primary motor cortex in children with autism. Human Brain Mapping. 2012. Available online at: http://onlinelibrary.wiley.com

[47] Cossu G, Boria S, Copioli C, Bracceschi R, Giuberti V, Santelli E, et al. Motor representation of actions in children with autism. PLoS ONE. 2012; 7:e44779

[48] Haswell CC, Izawa J, Dowell L, Mostofsky S, Shadmehr R. Representation of internal models of action in the autistic brain. Nature Neuroscience. 2009;**12**:970-972

[49] Hilton CL, Zhang Y, Whilte MR, Klohr CL, Constantino J. Motor impairment in sibling pairs concordant and discordant for ASDs. Autism. 2012; **16**(4):430-441

[50] Green D, Charman T, Pickles A, Chandler S, Loucas T, Simonoff E, et al. Impairment in movement skills of children with autistic spectrum disorders. Developmental Medicine and Child Neurology. 2009;**51**:311-316

[51] Dowell LR, Mahone EM, Mostofsky SH. Associations of postural knowledge

and basic motor skill with dyspraxia in autism: Implication for abnormalities in distributed connectivity and motor learning. Neuropsychology. 2009;**23**(5): 563-570

[52] Esposito G, Pasca SP. Motor abnormalities as a putative endophenotype for autism spectrum disorders. Frontiers in Integrative Neuroscience. 2013;**7**:43

[53] De Jong M, Punt M, De Groot E, Minderaa RB, Hadders-Algra M. Minor neurological dysfunction in children with autism spectrum disorder. Developmental Medicine and Child Neurology. 2011;**53**(7):641-646

[54] Freitag CM. The genetics of autistic disorders and its clinical relevance: A review of the literature. Molecular Psychiatry. 2007;**12**:2-22

[55] Chakrabarti S, Fombonne E. Pervasive developmental disorders in preschool children. JAMA. 2001;**285**: 3093-3099

[56] Wing L, Potter D. The epidemiology of autistic spectrum disorders: Is the prevalence rising. Mental Retardation and Developmental Disabilities Research Reviews. 2002;**8**:151-161

[57] CDC Centers for Disease Control and Prevention. Prevalence of autism spectrum disorders–Autism and developmental disabilities monitoring network. MMWR Surveillance Summaries. 2006;**58**:1-20

[58] Pinto-Martin JA, Levy SE, Feldman JF, Lorenz JM, Paneth N, Whitaker AH. Prevalence of autism spectrum disorder in adolescents born weighing <2000 grams. Pediatrics. 2011;**128**:883-891

[59] Movsas TZ, Paneth N. The effect of gestational age on symptom severity in children with autism spectrum disorder. Journal of Autism and Developmental Disorders. 2012;**42**:2431-2439

[60] Matson JL, Kozlowski AM. The increasing prevalence of autism spectrum disorders. Research in Autism Spectrum Disorder. 2011;**5**:418-425

[61] Kolevzon A, Gross R, Reichenberg A. Prenatal and perinatal risk factors for autism: A review and integration of findings. Archives of Pediatrics & Adolescent Medicine. 2007;**161**:326-333

[62] Schendel DE, Autry A, Wines R, Moore C. The co-occurrence of autism and birth defects: Prevalence and risk in a population-based cohort. Developmental Medicine and Child Neurology. 2009;**51**:779-786

[63] Williams K, Helmer M, Duncan GW, Peat JK, Mellis CM. Perinatal and maternal risk factors for autism spectrum disorders in New South Wales, Australia. Child: Care, Health and Development. 2008a;**34**:249-256

[64] Buchmayer S, Johansson S, Johansson A, Hultman CM, Sparen P, Cnattingius S. Can association between preterm birth and autism be explained by maternal or neonatal morbidity. Pediatrics. 2009;**124**:e817-e825

[65] Guinchat V, Thorsen P, Laurent C, Cans C, Bodeau N, Cohen D. Pre-, peri- and neonatal risk factors for autism. Acta Obstetricia et Gynecologica Scandinavica. 2012;**91**:287-300

[66] Lampi KM, Lehtonen L, Tran PL, Suominen A, Lehti V, Banerjee PN, et al. Risk of autism spectrum disorders in low birth weight and small for gestational age infants. The Journal of Pediatrics. 2012;**161**:830-836

[67] Kalkbrenner et al. Particulate matter exposure, prenatal and postnatal windows of susceptibility, and autism spectrum disorders. Epidemiology. 2015;**26**(1):30-42

[68] Dietert RR, Dietert JM, DeWitt JC. Environmental risk factors for autism.

Emerging Health Threats Journal. 2011; **4**:1-11

[69] Meldrum SJ, Strunk T, Currie A, Prescott SL, Simmer K, Whitehouse AJ. Autism spectrum disorder in children born preterm-role of exposure to perinatal inflammation. Frontiers in Neuroscience. 2013;**22**(7):123

[70] Goines PE, Ashwood P. Cytokine dysregulation in autism spectrum disorders (ASD): Possible role of the environment. Neurotoxicology and Teratology. 2013;**36**:67-81

[71] Morgan JT, Chana G, Pardo CA, Achim C, Semendeferi K, Buckwalter J, et al. Microglial activation and increased microglial density observed in the dorsolateral prefrontal cortex in autism. Biological Psychiatry. 2010;**68**:368-376

[72] Lintas C, Altieri L, Lombardi F, Sacco R, Persico AM. Association of autism with polyomavirus infection in postmortem brains. Journal of Neurovirology. 2010;**16**:141-149

[73] Groen SE et al. General movements in early infancy predict neuromotor development at 9 to 12 years of age. Developmental Medicine and Child Neurology. 2005;**47**(11):731-738

[74] Hadders-Algra M. General Movements: A window for early identification of children at high risk for developmental disorders. Journal of Pediatrics. 2004;**145**:S12-S18

[75] Burger et al. General movements as a predictive tool of the neurological outcome in very low and extremely low birth weight infants–A South African perspective. Early Human Development. 2011;**87**(4):303-308

[76] Harrison P, Oakland T. Adaptive Behavioral Assessment Scale. 2nd ed. San Antonio, Texas, USA: The Psychological Corporation; 2003

[77] Shapiro F. Eye Movement Desensitization and Reprocessing (EMDR). Basic Principles, Protocols and Procedures. 2nd ed. NY, USA: The Guilford Press; 2001

Section 6

Systems Biology Perspectives

Chapter 8

Systems Biology Perspectives for Studying Neurodevelopmental Events

Elodie Mathieux and Marco Antonio Mendoza-Parra

Abstract

Brain development follows a complex process orchestrated by diverse molecular and cellular events for which a perturbation can cause pathologies. In fact, multiple neuronal cell fate decisions driven by complex gene regulatory programs are involved in neurogenesis and neurodevelopment, and their characterization are part of the current challenges on neurobiology. In this chapter, we provide an overview of the various genomic strategies in use to explore the spatiotemporally defined gene regulatory wires implicated in brain development. Finally, we will discuss the intake of these approaches for understanding the multifactorial events implicated in neurodevelopment and the future requirements for further expanding our understanding of the brain.

Keywords: neurogenesis, gene regulatory networks, cell fate, systems biology, functional genomics

1. Introduction

Since the release of the first draft of the human genome and the development of massive parallel DNA sequencing strategies, our understanding of the genetic basis for a variety of human illnesses, including neurological disease, has expanded rapidly. In fact, around 50% of the known Mendelian disorders were already matched with their underlined genes [1] and this gap is expected to further decrease, namely by the improvements in the analysis of non-coding genomic regions [2]. This being said, the performance on the identification of the genetic context of diseases with complex phenotypes is more modest, probably due to their multigenic etiology. In fact, the use of exome sequencing for the detection of new mutations in an unknown gene in family pedigrees appeared as a straight approach in the context of Mendelian disorders, but at most it provides the list of common variants when applied to neurological illnesses with complex phenotypes. As a consequence, further functional genomic readouts, including transcriptomes, transcription factors profiling, or epigenetic landscaping, are required to further narrow the observed mutations and to reconstitute the complex relationship among the various genes implicated on the inset of the disease.

In this context, this chapter will focus on the use of such further readouts to complement previous exome sequencing efforts (for a review on the use of exome sequencing applied to neurological diseases: [3]) and provide an overview of the

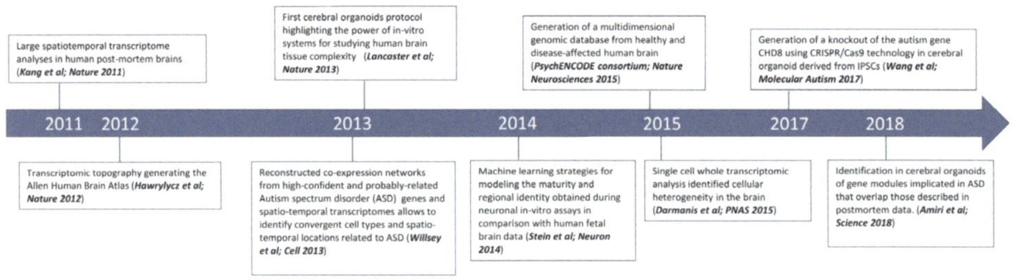

Figure 1.
Timeline recapitulating major achievements in understanding of healthy or disease-affected human brain development by the use of functional genomics approaches.

integrative computational strategies in use. Importantly, the concept of gene networks as an approach to describe the inter-relationship among the various implicated genes on the disease is discussed and illustrated by the major efforts performed over the last years in the field of neurodevelopment and related diseases (**Figure 1**). Finally, we discuss the arrival of new technological approaches for enhancing our capacity to interrogate the human nervous tissue, which in contrary to other tissues, remained till recently restricted to postmortem collected samples.

2. Interrogating neurodevelopment events by functional genomics

The evolution of genomics analyses, notably due to the sequencing of the human genome, allowed to study neurodevelopment from a different perspective; i.e., by the interrogation of the role of the genetic context during neurodevelopment. In fact, while the implication of genes in this process was previously studied at the individual level with the use of in-situ hybridization and RT-PCR methods, the developments in DNA microarray and RNA-sequencing technologies provided a global perspective as witnessed by the various studies focused on the brain transcriptome either from the whole organ or particular regions and across stages of development. Among them, the work, performed by Kang et al., for the establishment of transcriptomes from 57 postmortem human brains in 16 regions across the lifespan spanning developmental embryos through adulthood corresponds to one of the earliest most comprehensive studies. In fact, beyond the large amounts of data, they provided a spatiotemporal transcriptome regulation view enhanced by the establishment of gene co-expression networks recapitulating different stages of development. Importantly, this study highlighted that the majority of spatiotemporal differences happen before the birth with a shift of gene expression patterns around the birth in the neocortex. Principally in the fetal brain, genes with a role in cell proliferation, cell migration, and neuronal differentiation are expressed in contrast to the late fetal period and infancy, where genes coding to dendrite and synapse development are found [4].

Further studies performed by Colantuoni et al. focused on the temporal dynamic of the transcriptome in prefrontal cortex in a large number of human brain samples demonstrated that genes expressed differently in prenatal brain fetal development are reversed during postnatal life [5] with the recruitment of new genes in the early developmental brain [6]. With the same idea, the pattern of spatial gene expression in brain was shown to follow a way determined by embryonic origin that can change during development [7]. In fact, Pletikos et al. defined three phases in neocortical development: the prenatal with highest differential gene expression, the preadolescent phase with increasing synchronization of areal transcriptome, and the adolescence where differential expressions among area reappear [8]. The spatial part of transcriptome analysis gave the proof of structure gene regulation in human brain. Especially, differences in gene expression profiling were demonstrated between brain substructures or sites with the presence of region-specific genes [9–11]. Hawrylycz et al. combined histological analysis with microarray in 900 neuroanatomic subdivisions from two human brains and observed that the spatial topography of the neocortex is reflected in its transcriptomic topography where closer cortical regions have similar gene expression [12]. However, symmetry bilaterally between two hemispheres was observed during development [8, 9, 11]. In addition, the gene expression variability exists also between layers of neocortex. The neocortex consists of six horizontal layers with subsets of neurons, the transcriptional analysis of the layers in prefrontal cortex showed human specific layer gene expression patterns [13]. A study realized by Miller et al. demonstrated differential gene expression between proliferative and postmitotic layers in mid gestation human fetal brain with the presence of a molecular gradient frontotemporal in cortical layers [14]. These observations supported the gene expression gradients along the anteroposterior axis of neocortex [15].

While informative, the transcriptome analysis over the whole brain or performed on specific regions is issued from the analysis of multiple cells possibly presenting heterogeneous cell types populations. The development in single-cell transcriptomics appears as a relevant alternative for gathering information about cell types. The single-cell whole transcriptomic analysis permitted to identify cellular heterogeneity in the brain and subtypes of neuronal cells with differential gene expression between fetal and adult neurons [16]. Single nuclear transcriptome in the adult cerebral cortex was used to see diversity in neuronal subtypes and neuroanatomical areas [17]. Habib et al. combined this technique of single nucleus RNA-Seq with pulse-labeling proliferative cells using the thymidine analog, the 5-ethynyl-2′-deoxyuridine (EdU), to identify hippocampal cellular types and track transcriptional trajectories single proliferating cells in the adult hippocampal neurogenic niche [18]. Similarly, a recent single-cell RNA-Seq study in the human fetal cortex and medial ganglionic eminence during prenatal neurogenesis demonstrated the presence of lineage specific trajectories dependent of transcription regulatory [19]. This study also demonstrated the modest transcriptional differences in cortical radial glia cascade which conducts robust typological differences in neurons. In the same context, Lake et al. combined single-cell sequencing with epigenome readouts in adult human brain cells to reveal chromatin/transcription factor regulatory events within distinct cell types [20]. Recently, Fan et al. also performed single-cell spatial transcriptome analysis in human brain mid gestation embryos, where they observed heterogeneity in each cortex region with no synchronization in cortex development and maturation [21].

The study of the transcriptional expression behavior during brain development is expected to enhance our understanding of pathological situations. Autism spectrum disorder (ASD), a heterogeneous pathology with prevalence of 1 in 59 children, is one of these examples. The pathogenesis of ASD is characterized by social impairments, disrupted communication skills and repetitive behaviors. Numerous genes were shown to be implicated in ASD and their gene co-expression and/or gene regulatory networks analyses are providing new insights on the impaired/affected pathways on this disorder. In fact, several studies have tried to identify transcriptome alterations implicated in ASD using either DNA microarray hybridization assays or genome sequencing. By comparing autistic and control brain samples, upregulated genes implicated in immune function, while others repressed and involved in neurodevelopment or synaptogenesis were highlighted [22–24]. Another study described a dysregulation in mitochondrial oxidative phosphorylation and protein translation pathways without seeing changes in DNA methylation [25]. Consistent with this observation, the downregulation of genes involved in mitochondrial and synaptic function were also reported by using multiple genomics datasets like RNA-Seq and microarray studies previously published [26]. Interestingly, dysfunction in synaptic pathways was also described in another neurodevelopmental disease, namely schizophrenia [27–30]. This pathology affecting approximately 1% of the population is characterized by personality disturbances, hallucinations, delusions, and/or disorganizing behavior. High-throughput transcriptomic analysis revealed multiple deregulated genes in schizophrenia [29–32]. Several of them are implicated in neurodevelopmental pathways, neuronal communication, energy metabolism, and synaptic function [29, 30, 32]. Changes in DNA methylation related to the prenatal-postnatal life transition were also reported by comparing schizophrenia postmortem and unaffected control brain samples, strongly arguing for the implication of an epigenetic regulation in the disease's development [33–35].

In addition to the observed changes in gene expression, alternative RNA splicing has been described to occur at high frequency in human brain samples, corresponding to more than one-third of the human brain transcriptome [9, 36]. In addition, beyond the reported changes in protein coding gene expression [37], non-coding micro RNAs (miRNA) and/or long non-coding RNAs (lncRNA) were shown to have a role in neurodevelopment, participating in the reinforcement of brain complexity. Indeed, Ziats et al. described differential miRNAs expression in different parts of human brain along time of development with a principal shift that happens after the birth [38]. In the same idea, changes in lncRNA transcriptome during brain development [39], preferentially across fetal development with spatial regulation, were described [40]. LncRNAs also play a role in neuronal differentiation and neurogenesis, as suggested by studies highlighting a differential expression of lncRNAs during differentiation from human pluripotent stem cells [41, 42]. One example is the lncRNA rhabdomyosarcoma 2-associated transcript (RMST) which through its interaction with SOX2 regulates downstream genes implicated in neurogenesis [43]. The dysregulation of miRNA or lncRNA expression was also observed in autism [44–46], schizophrenia [47], and intellectual disability [48]. In this last case, lncRNAs were shown to be implicated in synaptic transmission, neurogenesis, or neurodevelopment.

Across these different transcriptome studies, a variety of databases hosting microarray and/or RNA-Seq data are currently available (for a comprehensive review, see [49]). Among them, we can cite the HB Atlas [4, 9], the BrainSpan Consortium [14], Brain Cloud [5], the Allen Brain map portal [12], the cortex single cells [19], or the single-cell portal [18]. In addition, several consortia, sometimes covering topics beyond the brain tissue, are at the basis of the establishment of major databases. Among others, we can cite the "Genotype Tissue Expression (GTex)" regrouping gene expression data issued from different tissues covering more than 600 donors [50]. Similarly, the "Encyclopedia of DNA Elements (ENCODE)" regroups large-scale datasets from various projects and combines multi-omics data from different species, variety of cell lines and tissues at different stages of development. A more specialized version of ENCODE, the "Psychiatric Encyclopedia of DNA Elements (PsychENCODE)," collects datasets concerning epigenetic modifications and non-coding RNA in healthy and disease-related human brains [51]. In the context of the data issued from brain samples, Huisman et al. developed the web portal "Brainscope" providing an interactive visualization of Allen Atlas adult brain transcriptome and across different stages of development [52]. Recently, a method to predict mRNA expression in whole brain using microarray data from Allen Brain Atlas with in-vivo positron emission tomography (PET) data was developed [53]. Overall, the generation of these databases correspond to major efforts for the research community, providing centralized access to the large collections of data; thus, further efforts of data integration can be performed, for instance by the reconstruction of gene regulatory networks on the basis of previously generated transcriptomes.

3. Inferring molecular coregulatory events from the integration of collected functional genomic readouts

The development of mid/high throughput strategies for analyzing genome sequences, their variants, gene expression, or even the proteome composition, provided means to the scientific community to interrogate each of these layers of complexity in a variety of model systems and tissues and in addition to integrate them to reconstruct a regulatory view. As illustrated in the previous section, several studies described major functional genomic readouts focused on studying brain development in normal and disease settings.

While being comprehensive, in most cases they provide relevant list of players (gene variants, differentially expressed genes, etc.) on the basis of statistical descriptors but forgets completely to address their potential relationship. Or, from a biological point of view, each of the players composing the system under study is expected to directly (or indirectly) influence the behavior of others. As a consequence, the current challenge is to evolve into an integrative view, focused on studying the various "deregulated events" as interconnected entities by the incorporation of multiple types of readouts and supported by computational solutions.

From an historical perspective, the article of Walsh et al. released in Science in 2008, corresponds to one of the first major studies aiming at identifying neurodevelopmental programs involved in a disease context like schizophrenia [54]. In this study, the authors hypothesized that the collective contribution of each of the rare structural variants retrieved on neurological/neurodevelopmental syndromes accounts for these disorders, and in the specific case of schizophrenia, they have demonstrated a difference of at least 3-fold between controls and individuals with schizophrenia on the frequency of rare structural variants within coding regions. Furthermore, they have focused on structural mutations that disrupt genes, and evaluated their functions with the help of computational solutions querying for gene enrichment in one or more functionally defined pathways (PANTHER and Ingenuity Pathway Analysis). This strategy per se aims at establishing gene relationships on the basis of their annotation to a given program (or pathway), even though in this case such relationships are inferred in-silico.

Since then, further studies incorporated other types of data, like the use of RNA-Seq transcriptomic analysis to identify the differentially expressed genes between controls and individuals with schizophrenia, which are then associated to biological functions by Gene ontology analysis [55–57]. Furthermore, the development of computational solutions for enhancing data integration has being performed like in the case of NETBAG, which allows to integrate multiple types of genetic variations like single nucleotide variants (SNVs), rare copy number variants (CNVs), and genome-wide association studies (GWAS), to identify highly connected gene clusters, potentially related to functional roles. NETBAG was initially described in the context of de novo CNVs in autism [58] and schizophrenia [59].

Beyond correlating changes in gene expression with the identification of genetic variations, further efforts are required for stratifying information, like the use of gene co-expression strategies. This approach aims at aggregating genes on the grounds of their expression levels under the hypothesis that co-expressed genes are the consequence of a common regulatory force; e.g., the action of transcription factors. This analysis can be represented under a network structure, on which a pair of genes is displayed interconnected on the basis of their significant co-expression relationship. This strategy has been applied by Voineagu and colleagues to resolve consistent differences in transcriptomes assessed over autistic and normal brain samples [23]. Specifically, they have resolved gene expression levels in cortical regions (suggesting cortical abnormalities in the context of autism), but in addition they have managed to identify discrete modules of co-expressed genes, clearly demonstrating the advantages of such strategy for enhancing the analytical resolution. Since then, various studies incorporated gene co-expression analysis together with genome-wide association data (GWAS) [60, 61], incorporated multiple human brain regions and issued from various human development stages as a way to identify specific biological processes and defined brain regions associated to autism disorder [62, 63].

While gene co-expression networks are expected to be the consequence of the action of defined master transcription factors, their identity remains unknown in this type of analysis. The combination of chromatin immunoprecipitation (ChIP) with massive parallel sequencing provided means to scrutinize the genome locations on which given TFs are located. Furthermore, on the basis of their proximity to annotated coding regions, it is possible to infer their transcriptional regulation activity over proximal genes. Following such strategy, factors like TBR1 [64] or Auts2 [65, 66], initially identified by rare genetic variant studies were ChIP-sequenced to reveal their direct targets. In both cases, they were found located on genomic regions adjacent to autism spectrum disorder (ASD)-related genes. A similar strategy has been applied to map the gene targets associated to the chromatin modifier CHD8 (chromodomain helicase) [67], previously shown to be mutated in rare genetic variant studies [68].

Although powerful for the identification of the target genes for a given factor, performing ChIP-Seq assays remains still challenging for covering a large number of TFs, epigenetic modifications, and/or chromatin remodelers which could appear associated to neurodevelopmental events. In fact, identifying strategies to prioritize the list of TFs to be immunoprecipitated remains a key step, which is currently handled by applying computational strategies. In this context, we have recently developed TETRAMER, a computational approach able to reconstruct gene regulatory networks from the integration of transcriptomes provided by the user and annotations retrieved in various databases concerning TF-Target gene relationships [69]. Furthermore, TETRAMER simulates transcription regulation propagation over the reconstructed connectivity to identify master TFs, which could then be prioritized for experimental assays. This strategy has been initially used for identifying novel master TFs implicated on neurogenesis by reconstructing gene regulatory networks from temporal transcriptomes [70]; then, it has been extrapolated to a collection of more than 3000 transcriptomes covering ~300 cell/tissue types and representing 14 different anatomical systems in the human body. Among them, 58 cell/tissue types composing the human nervous system were analyzed, for which their relevant master TFs as well as their related gene regulatory networks were inferred. As illustrated in **Figure 2**, this type of analysis allows to compare the fraction of shared TFs retrieved on different nervous systems, thus providing to highlight relevant players implicated on their transcriptional regulation. In **Figure 2**, a comparison between the TFs retrieved on frontal cortex and hypothalamus is depicted, revealing the presence of factors like TBR1 or ARNT2, previously identified as presenting rare genetic variants associated to autism disorders [64, 71] or NPAS3, previously described as a master regulator of neuropsychiatric related genes [72].

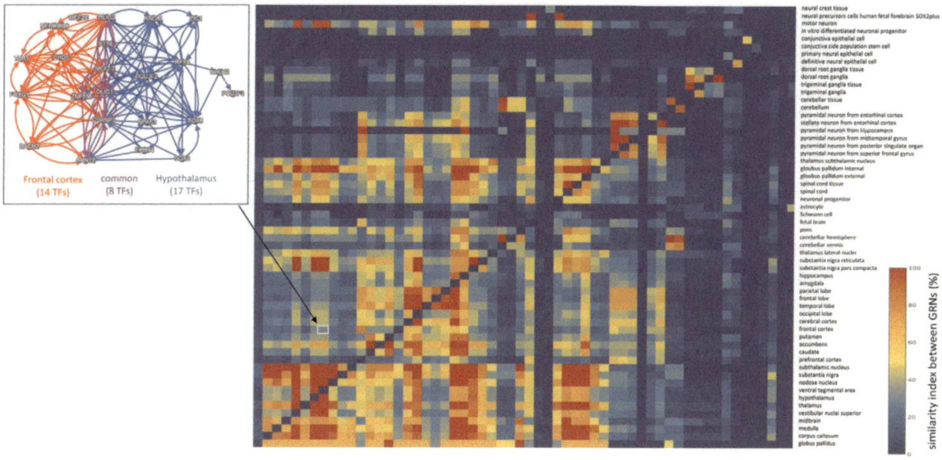

Figure 2.
Comparison of 58 nervous system cell/tissue types on the basis of their master TF co-regulatory networks. The fraction of common TFs pairwise is displayed in percentage (heatmap). The inset displays the identity of the major TFs retrieved in Frontal cortex compared with those retrieved on hypothalamus. The illustrated data are extracted from the analysis performed over more than 3000 Affymetrix arrays corresponding to ~300 cell/tissue types describing 14 different systems on the human body (Cholley et al. [69]).

Overall, the analytical strategies aforementioned clearly suggest the necessity of incorporating various types of genetic and functional genomic readouts such that their inter-relationship might enhance our comprehension of the phenomena under study. This is more relevant when studying neurodevelopment and their related diseases as the consequence of multigenetic events. Furthermore, it is important to mention that data integration is systematically supported by computational developments, as witnessed by the various tools and computational strategies devoted to infer relationships among the available data, but also to model systems behavior. Notably, the use of machine learning strategies for modeling the maturity and regional identity obtained during neuronal in-vitro assays in comparison with human fetal brain data, provide means to take advantage of in-vitro systems that manage to reconstitute as close as possible the in-vivo events [73]. In a similar manner, major efforts like the "blue brain project" are currently combining data assessment with computational modeling to reconstruct cell atlas for instance of the mouse brain [74], strongly suggesting that over the coming years major discoveries in neuroscience might arise from such multidisciplinary efforts.

4. Perspectives for the coming years: from the use of new in-vitro 3D-brain tissue models, single cell strategies to big-data systems biology

The majority of transcriptome or related studies in human brain used postmortem tissues as source of material. As consequence, technical concerns like the potential RNA degradation following pre- and postmortem factors as environment, collection methods, or postmortem interval could directly influence the quality of the readouts [75–77]. The use of animal models as an alternative is losing interest due to the reported differences, for instance in human corticogenesis relative to mouse models, which are further supported by human specific gene signature and/or divergences in gene regulatory programs [78–80]. Even if few percentages of genes have different trajectories in non-human primate and human in contrast to rodent, this model can help to understand brain development, but it cannot model all features found in human [79, 81]. In fact, comparison between non-human primate and human brains transcriptome analysis showed human specificity in gene expression profiling [82–84] with demonstration that genes differentially expressed are principally upregulated in human brains in contrast to other organs [85, 86]. In addition, the transcriptome remodeling during postnatal periods appears delayed in human brain comparing to non-human primate [87].

More recently, the use of human-induced pluripotent stem cells (hIPSCs) combined with in-vitro culture strategies for generating two- or three-dimensional nervous tissue appears as an alternative to animal model systems. In fact, nowadays it is possible to generate hIPSCs from tissue samples collected from patients presenting neurological disorders which can be differentiated toward nervous tissue. In this context, a recent study compared the transcriptome of neural stem cells driven in-vitro toward corticogenesis and discovered a strong conservation with in-vivo gene expression with the conservation of cortical gene network implicated in ASD [73]. In contrast to the in-vitro neuronal differentiation in two dimensions, the generation of three-dimensional models (known as cerebral organoids) appears as a more relevant physiological model to study neurodevelopment [88–91]. Comparing human cerebral organoids and fetal brain development demonstrated the similarity in gene expression programs and epigenomic signatures [92–94]. Furthermore, single-cell transcriptome analysis over cerebral organoids revealed an important cellular heterogeneity, reminiscent to what is observed in the human brain [95]. As a consequence, the use of human cerebral organoids corresponds to a new approach for modeling the neuronal development and providing means to study neurogenesis from a systems biology perspective. For example, Mariani et al. generated cerebral organoids from hIPSCs derived from patients with ASD and recapitulated transcriptional programs present in fetal cortical development. In this study, the use of gene network analyses allowed to identify upregulated gene programs implicated in cell proliferation, neuronal differentiation and synaptic process [90]. Similarly, Amiri et al. identified gene modules implicated in ASD that overlap those described previously in postmortem data. This study supported the idea that cerebral organoids provide means to reveal gene regulatory elements contributing to ASD [94]. Due to these success, major efforts focused on the development of protocols to generate tissues reminiscent to different brain structures like forebrain [90, 96], midbrain [96, 97], or hypothalamus [96] were developed. Recently, chimeric organoids issued from the fusion different regionalized organoids (like dorsal-ventral forebrain organoids) were generated to increase the complexity of the generated tissues [98].

The use of cerebral organoids as a model system for studying neurodevelopment and related diseases is in its infancy. This approach still requires improvements, for instance in the context of the reproducibility, but due to its alternative to human postmortem samples and animal models, it is expected to continue to evolve over the coming years. In fact, this tendency is also boosted by multiple other developments, including the use of CRISPR/CAS9 system to engineer organoids [99], the democratization of single cell omics strategies [95], as well as the gain in multidisciplinary approaches, specifically by the incorporation of computational approaches for modeling brain tissue organization [74].

5. Conclusion

Understanding the brain complexity corresponds to one of the major challenges for the scientific community. This does not only imply its physiological function, but also its relationship with the human mind. The use of omics strategies is revolutionizing the way to interpret any living system from the expression of their genome, and in the particular case of the human brain, it is enhancing the comprehension of neurological disorders. In this chapter, we have discussed the use of transcriptomes, exome sequencing, and gene regulatory network strategies for revealing the influence of multiple genes. Furthermore, we have highlighted the arrival of cerebral organoids as a novel model system for studying human nervous system, which in combination with further developments (single-cell strategies, CRISPR-Cas9 engineering, etc.) is a promising major progress for understanding the brain function. This enthusiasm is further supported with the major advancements in computational developments, notably the artificial intelligence, which together with the major amounts of data (issued from omics strategies) is expected to accelerate discoveries. Overall, we expect that this chapter will open the mind to young readers to further explore the multidisciplinary approaches described herein to directly participate in the exploration of the human brain in the following years.

Acknowledgements

We thank all members of the SysFate lab for discussions related to the elaboration of this chapter. SysFate is supported by the "Genopole Thematic Incentive Actions" funding (referred to by their French acronym "ATIGE") and by the institutional bodies CEA, CNRS, and Université d'Evry, Université Paris-Saclay.

Conflict of interest

The authors declare that there is no conflict of interest.

Nomenclature

DNA	deoxyribonucleic acid
RT-PCR	reverse transcription polymerase chain reaction
RNA	ribonucleic acid
RNA-Seq	RNA sequencing
EdU	5-ethynyl-2′-deoxyuridine
ASD	autism spectrum disorder
miRNA	micro-RNA
lncRNA	long non-coding RNA
RMST	rhabdomyosarcoma 2-associated transcript
SOX2	sex determining region Y-box 2
GTex	genotype tissue expression
ENCODE	encyclopedia of DNA elements
PsychENCODE	psychiatric encyclopedia of DNA elements
PET	positron emission tomography
SNV	single nucleotide variants
CNV	copy number variants
GWAS	genome-wide association studies
ChIP	chromatin immunoprecipitation
TF	transcription factor
TBR1	T-box, brain 1
Auts2	activator of transcription and developmental regulator
CHD8	chromodomain helicase DNA binding protein 8

ARNT2	aryl hydrocarbon receptor nuclear translocator 2
NPAS3	neuronal PAS domain protein 3
hIPSCs	human-induced pluripotent stem cells
CRISPR/CAS9	clustered regularly interspaced short palindromic repeats/CRISPR-associated 9
Transcriptome	total of RNA molecules expressed in a cell or a population of cells
Exome	the part of the genome composed of exons which are the coding portions of gene
Epigenome	multitude of chemical compounds and proteins that modify and control the expression of genes without change in DNA sequence
MicroRNA	class of small non-coding RNA molecules of about 22 nucleotides in length that function as posttranscriptional regulators of target genes
LncRNA	non-coding RNA molecules greater than 200 nucleotides in length
Single nucleotide variants	loci with alleles that differ at a single base
Rare copy number variants	number of copies of a particular gene that varies between individuals
Genome-wide association study (GWAS)	approach to associate specific genetic variations with particular diseases
Chromatin immunoprecipitation	procedure to investigate interaction between proteins and genomic DNA regions

Author details

Elodie Mathieux and Marco Antonio Mendoza-Parra*
Génomique Métabolique, Genoscope, Institut François Jacob, CEA, CNRS, Univ Evry, Université Paris-Saclay, Evry, France

*Address all correspondence to: mmendoza@genoscope.cns.fr

References

[1] Chong JX, Buckingham KJ, Jhangiani SN, Boehm C, Sobreira N, Smith JD, et al. The genetic basis of mendelian phenotypes: Discoveries, challenges, and opportunities. American Journal of Human Genetics. 2015;**97**(2):199-215

[2] Kremer LS, Bader DM, Mertes C, Kopajtich R, Pichler G, Iuso A, et al. Genetic diagnosis of Mendelian disorders via RNA sequencing. Nature Communications. 2017;**8**:15824

[3] Keogh MJ, Chinnery PF. Next generation sequencing for neurological diseases: New hope or new hype? Clinical Neurology and Neurosurgery. 2013;**115**(7):948-953

[4] Kang HJ, Kawasawa YI, Cheng F, Zhu Y, Xu X, Li M, et al. Spatio-temporal transcriptome of the human brain. Nature. 2011;**478**(7370):483-489

[5] Colantuoni C, Lipska BK, Ye T, Hyde TM, Tao R, Leek JT, et al. Temporal dynamics and genetic control of transcription in the human prefrontal cortex. Nature. 2011;**478**(7370):519-523

[6] Zhang YE, Landback P, Vibranovski MD, Long M. Accelerated recruitment of new brain development genes into the human genome. PLoS Biology. 2011; **9**(10):e1001179

[7] Kirsch L, Chechik G. On expression patterns and developmental origin of human brain regions. PLoS Computational Biology. 2016;**12**(8): e1005064

[8] Pletikos M, Sousa AMM, Sedmak G, Meyer KA, Zhu Y, Cheng F, et al. Temporal specification and bilaterality of human neocortical topographic gene expression. Neuron. 2014;**81**(2):321-332

[9] Johnson MB, Kawasawa YI, Mason CE, Krsnik Z, Coppola G, Bogdanović D, et al. Functional and evolutionary insights into human brain development through global transcriptome analysis. Neuron. 2009;**62**(4):494-509

[10] Roth RB, Hevezi P, Lee J, Willhite D, Lechner SM, Foster AC, et al. Gene expression analyses reveal molecular relationships among 20 regions of the human CNS. Neurogenetics. 2006;**7**(2): 67-80

[11] Lambert N, Lambot M-A, Bilheu A, Albert V, Englert Y, Libert F, et al. Genes expressed in specific areas of the human fetal cerebral cortex display distinct patterns of evolution. PLoS One. 2011;**6**(3):e17753

[12] Hawrylycz MJ, Lein ES, Guillozet-Bongaarts AL, Shen EH, Ng L, Miller JA, et al. An anatomically comprehensive atlas of the adult human brain transcriptome. Nature. 2012;**489**(7416): 391-399

[13] He Z, Han D, Efimova O, Guijarro P, Yu Q, Oleksiak A, et al. Comprehensive transcriptome analysis of neocortical layers in humans, chimpanzees and macaques. Nature Neuroscience. 2017;**20**(6):886-895

[14] Miller JA, Ding S-L, Sunkin SM, Smith KA, Ng L, Szafer A, et al. Transcriptional landscape of the prenatal human brain. Nature. 2014; **508**(7495):199-206

[15] Ip BK, Wappler I, Peters H, Lindsay S, Clowry GJ, Bayatti N. Investigating gradients of gene expression involved in early human cortical development. Journal of Anatomy. 2010;**217**(4):300-311

[16] Darmanis S, Sloan SA, Zhang Y, Enge M, Caneda C, Shuer LM, et al. A survey of human brain transcriptome diversity at the single cell level. Proceedings of the National Academy of Sciences of the United States of America. 2015;**112**(23):7285-7290

[17] Lake BB, Ai R, Kaeser GE, Salathia NS, Yung YC, Liu R, et al. Neuronal subtypes and diversity revealed by single-nucleus RNA sequencing of the human brain. Science. 2016;**352**(6293): 1586-1590

[18] Habib N, Li Y, Heidenreich M, Swiech L, Avraham-Davidi I, Trombetta JJ, et al. Div-Seq: Single-nucleus RNA-Seq reveals dynamics of rare adult newborn neurons. Science. 2016; **353**(6302):925-928

[19] Nowakowski TJ, Bhaduri A, Pollen AA, Alvarado B, Mostajo-Radji MA, Di Lullo E, et al. Spatiotemporal gene expression trajectories reveal developmental hierarchies of the human cortex. Science. 2017;**358**(6368): 1318-1323

[20] Lake BB, Chen S, Sos BC, Fan J, Kaeser GE, Yung YC, et al. Integrative single-cell analysis of transcriptional and epigenetic states in the human adult brain. Nature Biotechnology. 2018; **36**(1):70-80

[21] Fan X, Dong J, Zhong S, Wei Y, Wu Q, Yan L, et al. Spatial transcriptomic survey of human embryonic cerebral cortex by single-cell RNA-seq analysis. Cell Research. 2018;**28**(7):730-745

[22] Garbett K, Ebert PJ, Mitchell A, Lintas C, Manzi B, Mirnics K, et al. Immune transcriptome alterations in the temporal cortex of subjects with autism. Neurobiology of Disease. 2008;**30**(3): 303-311

[23] Voineagu I, Wang X, Johnston P, Lowe JK, Tian Y, Horvath S, et al. Transcriptomic analysis of autistic brain reveals convergent molecular pathology. Nature. 2011;**474**(7351):380-384

[24] Chow ML, Pramparo T, Winn ME, Barnes CC, Li H-R, Weiss L, et al. Age-dependent brain gene expression and copy number anomalies in autism suggest distinct pathological processes at young versus mature ages. PLoS Genetics. 2012;**8**(3):e1002592

[25] Ginsberg MR, Rubin RA, Falcone T, Ting AH, Natowicz MR. Brain transcriptional and epigenetic associations with autism. PLoS One. 2012;7(9):e44736

[26] Schwede M, Nagpal S, Gandal MJ, Parikshak NN, Mirnics K, Geschwind DH, et al. Strong correlation of downregulated genes related to synaptic transmission and mitochondria in post-mortem autism cerebral cortex. Journal of Neurodevelopmental Disorders. 2018;**10**(1):18

[27] Ellis SE, Panitch R, West AB, Arking DE. Transcriptome analysis of cortical tissue reveals shared sets of downregulated genes in autism and schizophrenia. Translational Psychiatry. 2016;**6**:e817

[28] Jaffe AE, Straub RE, Shin JH, Tao R, Gao Y, Collado-Torres L, et al. Developmental and genetic regulation of the human cortex transcriptome illuminate schizophrenia pathogenesis. Nature Neuroscience. 2018;**21**(8): 1117-1125

[29] Mistry M, Gillis J, Pavlidis P. Genome-wide expression profiling of schizophrenia using a large combined cohort. Molecular Psychiatry. 2013; **18**(2):215-225

[30] Mudge J, Miller NA, Khrebtukova I, Lindquist IE, May GD, Huntley JJ, et al. Genomic convergence analysis of schizophrenia: mRNA sequencing reveals altered synaptic vesicular transport in post-mortem cerebellum. PLoS One. 2008;**3**(11):e3625

[31] Cohen OS, Mccoy SY, Middleton FA, Bialosuknia S, Zhang-James Y, Liu L, et al. Transcriptomic analysis of postmortem brain identifies dysregulated splicing events in novel

candidate genes for schizophrenia. Schizophrenia Research. 2012;**142**(1–3): 188-199

[32] Pérez-Santiago J, Diez-Alarcia R, Callado LF, Zhang JX, Chana G, White CH, et al. A combined analysis of microarray gene expression studies of the human prefrontal cortex identifies genes implicated in schizophrenia. Journal of Psychiatric Research. 2012; **46**(11):1464-1474

[33] Jaffe AE, Gao Y, Deep-Soboslay A, Tao R, Hyde TM, Weinberger DR, et al. Mapping DNA methylation across development, genotype and schizophrenia in the human frontal cortex. Nature Neuroscience. 2016;**19**(1):40-47

[34] Numata S, Ye T, Herman M, Lipska BK. DNA methylation changes in the postmortem dorsolateral prefrontal cortex of patients with schizophrenia. Frontiers in Genetics. 2014;**5**:280

[35] Hannon E, Spiers H, Viana J, Pidsley R, Burrage J, Murphy TM, et al. Methylation QTLs in the developing brain and their enrichment in schizophrenia risk loci. Nature Neuroscience. 2016;**19**(1):48-54

[36] Mazin P, Xiong J, Liu X, Yan Z, Zhang X, Li M, et al. Widespread splicing changes in human brain development and aging. Molecular Systems Biology. 2013;**9**:633

[37] Myers AJ, Gibbs JR, Webster JA, Rohrer K, Zhao A, Marlowe L, et al. A survey of genetic human cortical gene expression. Nature Genetics. 2007; **39**(12):1494-1499

[38] Ziats MN, Rennert OM. Identification of differentially expressed microRNAs across the developing human brain. Molecular Psychiatry. 2014;**19**(7):848-852

[39] Lipovich L, Tarca AL, Cai J, Jia H, Chugani HT, Sterner KN, et al. Developmental changes in the transcriptome of human cerebral cortex tissue: Long noncoding RNA transcripts. Cerebral Cortex (New York, N.Y. : 1991). 2014;**24**(6):1451-1459

[40] Zhang X-Q, Wang Z-L, Poon M-W, Yang J-H. Spatial-temporal transcriptional dynamics of long non-coding RNAs in human brain. Human Molecular Genetics. 2017;**26**(16): 3202-3211

[41] Ng S-Y, Johnson R, Stanton LW. Human long non-coding RNAs promote pluripotency and neuronal differentiation by association with chromatin modifiers and transcription factors. The EMBO Journal. 2012;**31**(3): 522-533

[42] Lin M, Pedrosa E, Shah A, Hrabovsky A, Maqbool S, Zheng D, et al. RNA-Seq of human neurons derived from iPS cells reveals candidate long non-coding RNAs involved in neurogenesis and neuropsychiatric disorders. PLoS One. 2011;**6**(9):e23356

[43] Ng S-Y, Bogu GK, Soh BS, Stanton LW. The long noncoding RNA RMST interacts with SOX2 to regulate neurogenesis. Molecular Cell. 2013; **51**(3):349-359

[44] Abu-Elneel K, Liu T, Gazzaniga FS, Nishimura Y, Wall DP, Geschwind DH, et al. Heterogeneous dysregulation of microRNAs across the autism spectrum. Neurogenetics. 2008;**9**(3):153-161

[45] Ziats MN, Rennert OM. Aberrant expression of long noncoding RNAs in autistic brain. Journal of Molecular Neuroscience: MN. 2013;**49**(3):589-593

[46] Parikshak NN, Swarup V, Belgard TG, Irimia M, Ramaswami G, Gandal MJ, et al. Genome-wide changes in lncRNA, splicing, and regional gene expression patterns in autism. Nature. 2016;**540**(7633):423-427

[47] Perkins DO, Jeffries CD, Jarskog LF, Thomson JM, Woods K, Newman MA, et al. microRNA expression in the prefrontal cortex of individuals with schizophrenia and schizoaffective disorder. Genome Biology. 2007;**8**(2): R27

[48] D'haene E, Jacobs EZ, Volders P-J, De Meyer T, Menten B, Vergult S. Identification of long non-coding RNAs involved in neuronal development and intellectual disability. Scientific Reports. 2016;**6**:28396

[49] Keil JM, Qalieh A, Kwan KY. Brain transcriptome databases: A user's guide. Journal of Neuroscience: The Official Journal of the Society for Neuroscience. Mar 7, 2018;**38**(10):2399-2412

[50] GTEx Consortium. Human genomics. The genotype-tissue expression (GTEx) pilot analysis: Multitissue gene regulation in humans. Science. 2015;**348**(6235):648-660

[51] PsychENCODE Consortium, Akbarian S, Liu C, Knowles JA, Vaccarino FM, Farnham PJ, et al. The PsychENCODE project. Nature Neuroscience. 2015;**18**(12):1707-1712

[52] Huisman SMH, van Lew B, Mahfouz A, Pezzotti N, Höllt T, Michielsen L, et al. BrainScope: Interactive visual exploration of the spatial and temporal human brain transcriptome. Nucleic Acids Research. 2017;**45**(10):e83

[53] Gryglewski G, Seiger R, James GM, Godbersen GM, Komorowski A, Unterholzner J, et al. Spatial analysis and high resolution mapping of the human whole-brain transcriptome for integrative analysis in neuroimaging. NeuroImage. 2018;**176**:259-267

[54] Walsh T, McClellan JM, McCarthy SE, Addington AM, Pierce SB, Cooper GM, et al. Rare structural variants disrupt multiple genes in neurodevelopmental pathways in schizophrenia. Science. 2008;**320**(5875): 539-543

[55] Duan J, Sanders AR, Moy W, Drigalenko EI, Brown EC, Freda J, et al. Transcriptome outlier analysis implicates schizophrenia susceptibility genes and enriches putatively functional rare genetic variants. Human Molecular Genetics. 2015;**24**(16):4674-4685

[56] Sanders AR, Göring HHH, Duan J, Drigalenko EI, Moy W, Freda J, et al. Transcriptome study of differential expression in schizophrenia. Human Molecular Genetics. 2013;**22**(24): 5001-5014

[57] Wu JQ, Wang X, Beveridge NJ, Tooney PA, Scott RJ, Carr VJ, et al. Transcriptome sequencing revealed significant alteration of cortical promoter usage and splicing in schizophrenia. PLoS One. 2012;**7**(4): e36351

[58] Gilman SR, Iossifov I, Levy D, Ronemus M, Wigler M, Vitkup D. Rare de novo variants associated with autism implicate a large functional network of genes involved in formation and function of synapses. Neuron. 2011; **70**(5):898-907

[59] Gilman SR, Chang J, Xu B, Bawa TS, Gogos JA, Karayiorgou M, et al. Diverse types of genetic variation converge on functional gene networks involved in schizophrenia. Nature Neuroscience. 2012;**15**(12):1723-1728

[60] Ben-David E, Shifman S. Networks of neuronal genes affected by common and rare variants in autism spectrum disorders. PLoS Genetics. 2012;**8**(3): e1002556

[61] Ben-David E, Shifman S. Combined analysis of exome sequencing points toward a major role for transcription regulation during brain development in autism. Molecular Psychiatry. 2013; **18**(10):1054-1056

[62] Willsey AJ, Sanders SJ, Li M, Dong S, Tebbenkamp AT, Muhle RA, et al. Coexpression networks implicate human midfetal deep cortical projection neurons in the pathogenesis of autism. Cell. 2013;**155**(5):997-1007

[63] Parikshak NN, Luo R, Zhang A, Won H, Lowe JK, Chandran V, et al. Integrative functional genomic analyses implicate specific molecular pathways and circuits in autism. Cell. 2013;**155**(5): 1008-1021

[64] Notwell JH, Heavner WE, Darbandi SF, Katzman S, McKenna WL, Ortiz-Londono CF, et al. TBR1 regulates autism risk genes in the developing neocortex. Genome Research. 2016; **26**(8):1013-1022

[65] Oksenberg N, Haliburton GDE, Eckalbar WL, Oren I, Nishizaki S, Murphy K, et al. Genome-wide distribution of Auts2 binding localizes with active neurodevelopmental genes. Translational Psychiatry. 2014;**4**:e431

[66] Gao Z, Lee P, Stafford JM, von Schimmelmann M, Schaefer A, Reinberg D. An AUTS2-Polycomb complex activates gene expression in the CNS. Nature. 2014;**516**(7531):349-354

[67] Cotney J, Muhle RA, Sanders SJ, Liu L, Willsey AJ, Niu W, et al. The autism-associated chromatin modifier CHD8 regulates other autism risk genes during human neurodevelopment. Nature Communications. 2015;**6**:6404

[68] Bernier R, Golzio C, Xiong B, Stessman H, Coe BP, Penn O, et al. Disruptive CHD8 mutations define a subtype of autism early in development. Cell. 2014;**158**(2):263-276

[69] Cholley P-E, Moehlin J, Rohmer A, Zilliox V, Nicaise S, Gronemeyer H, et al. Modeling gene-regulatory networks to describe cell fate transitions and predict master regulators. NPJ Systems Biology and Applications. 2018; **4**(1):29

[70] Mendoza-Parra M-A, Malysheva V, Mohamed Saleem MA, Lieb M, Godel A, Gronemeyer H. Reconstructed cell fate-regulatory programs in stem cells reveal hierarchies and key factors of neurogenesis. Genome Research. 2016; **26**(11):1505-1519

[71] Di Napoli A, Warrier V, Baron-Cohen S, Chakrabarti B. Genetic variant rs17225178 in the ARNT2 gene is associated with Asperger Syndrome. Molecular Autism. 2015;**6**(1):9

[72] Michaelson JJ, Shin M-K, Koh J-Y, Brueggeman L, Zhang A, Katzman A, et al. Neuronal PAS domain proteins 1 and 3 are master regulators of neuropsychiatric risk genes. Biological Psychiatry. 2017;**82**(3):213-223

[73] Stein JL, de la Torre-Ubieta L, Tian Y, Parikshak NN, Hernández IA, Marchetto MC, et al. A quantitative framework to evaluate modeling of cortical development by neural stem cells. Neuron. 2014;**83**(1):69-86

[74] Erö C, Gewaltig M-O, Keller D, Markram H. A cell atlas for the mouse brain. Frontiers in Neuroinformatics. 2018;**12**:84

[75] Birdsill AC, Walker DG, Lue L, Sue LI, Beach TG. Postmortem interval effect on RNA and gene expression in human brain tissue. Cell and Tissue Banking. 2011;**12**(4):311-318

[76] Lipska BK, Deep-Soboslay A, Weickert CS, Hyde TM, Martin CE, Herman MM, et al. Critical factors in gene expression in postmortem human brain: Focus on studies in schizophrenia. Biological Psychiatry. 2006;**60**(6): 650-658

[77] Trabzuni D, Ryten M, Walker R, Smith C, Imran S, Ramasamy A, et al. Quality control parameters on a large

dataset of regionally dissected human control brains for whole genome expression studies. Journal of Neurochemistry. 2011;**119**(2):275-282

[78] Zeng H, Shen EH, Hohmann JG, Oh SW, Bernard A, Royall JJ, et al. Large-scale cellular-resolution gene profiling in human neocortex reveals species-specific molecular signatures. Cell. 2012; **149**(2):483-496

[79] Bakken TE, Miller JA, Ding S-L, Sunkin SM, Smith KA, Ng L, et al. A comprehensive transcriptional map of primate brain development. Nature. 2016;**535**(7612):367-375

[80] Wang P, Zhao D, Rockowitz S, Zheng D. Divergence and rewiring of regulatory networks for neural development between human and other species. Neurogenesis (Austin, TX). 2016;**3**(1):e1231495

[81] Bernard A, Lubbers LS, Tanis KQ, Luo R, Podtelezhnikov AA, Finney EM, et al. Transcriptional architecture of the primate neocortex. Neuron. 2012;**73**(6): 1083-1099

[82] Konopka G, Friedrich T, Davis-Turak J, Winden K, Oldham MC, Gao F, et al. Human-specific transcriptional networks in the brain. Neuron. 2012; **75**(4):601-617

[83] Sousa AMM, Zhu Y, Raghanti MA, Kitchen RR, Onorati M, Tebbenkamp ATN, et al. Molecular and cellular reorganization of neural circuits in the human lineage. Science. 2017; **358**(6366):1027-1032

[84] Xu C, Li Q, Efimova O, He L, Tatsumoto S, Stepanova V, et al. Human-specific features of spatial gene expression and regulation in eight brain regions. Genome Research. 2018;**28**(8): 1097-1110

[85] Khaitovich P, Muetzel B, She X, Lachmann M, Hellmann I, Dietzsch J, et al. Regional patterns of gene expression in human and chimpanzee brains. Genome Research. 2004;**14**(8): 1462-1473

[86] Cáceres M, Lachuer J, Zapala MA, Redmond JC, Kudo L, Geschwind DH, et al. Elevated gene expression levels distinguish human from non-human primate brains. Proceedings of the National Academy of Sciences of the United States of America. 2003;**100**(22): 13030-13035

[87] Somel M, Franz H, Yan Z, Lorenc A, Guo S, Giger T, et al. Transcriptional neoteny in the human brain. Proceedings of the National Academy of Sciences of the United States of America. 2009;**106**(14):5743-5748

[88] Lancaster MA, Renner M, Martin C-A, Wenzel D, Bicknell LS, Hurles ME, et al. Cerebral organoids model human brain development and microcephaly. Nature. 2013;**501**(7467):373-379

[89] Renner M, Lancaster MA, Bian S, Choi H, Ku T, Peer A, et al. Self-organized developmental patterning and differentiation in cerebral organoids. The EMBO Journal. 2017; **36**(10):1316-1329

[90] Mariani J, Coppola G, Zhang P, Abyzov A, Provini L, Tomasini L, et al. FOXG1-dependent dysregulation of GABA/glutamate neuron differentiation in autism spectrum disorders. Cell. 2015; **162**(2):375-390

[91] Matsui TK, Matsubayashi M, Sakaguchi YM, Hayashi RK, Zheng C, Sugie K, et al. Six-month cultured cerebral organoids from human ES cells contain matured neural cells. Neuroscience Letters. 2018;**670**:75-82

[92] Camp JG, Badsha F, Florio M, Kanton S, Gerber T, Wilsch-Bräuninger M, et al. Human cerebral organoids recapitulate gene expression programs of fetal neocortex development.

Proceedings of the National Academy of Sciences of the United States of America. 2015;**112**(51):15672-15677

[93] Luo C, Lancaster MA, Castanon R, Nery JR, Knoblich JA, Ecker JR. Cerebral organoids recapitulate epigenomic signatures of the human fetal brain. Cell Reports. 2016;**17**(12):3369-3384

[94] Amiri A, Coppola G, Scuderi S, Wu F, Roychowdhury T, Liu F, et al. Transcriptome and epigenome landscape of human cortical development modeled in organoids. Science. 2018;**362**(6420):14

[95] Quadrato G, Nguyen T, Macosko EZ, Sherwood JL, Min Yang S, Berger DR, et al. Cell diversity and network dynamics in photosensitive human brain organoids. Nature. 2017; **545**(7652):48-53

[96] Qian X, Nguyen HN, Song MM, Hadiono C, Ogden SC, Hammack C, et al. Brain-region-specific organoids using mini-bioreactors for modeling ZIKV exposure. Cell. 2016;**165**(5): 1238-1254

[97] Jo J, Xiao Y, Sun AX, Cukuroglu E, Tran H-D, Göke J, et al. Midbrain-like organoids from human pluripotent stem cells contain functional dopaminergic and neuromelanin-producing neurons. Cell Stem Cell. 2016;**19**(2):248-257

[98] Bagley JA, Reumann D, Bian S, Lévi-Strauss J, Knoblich JA. Fused cerebral organoids model interactions between brain regions. Nature Methods. 2017;**14**(7):743-751

[99] Wang P, Mokhtari R, Pedrosa E, Kirschenbaum M, Bayrak C, Zheng D, et al. CRISPR/Cas9-mediated heterozygous knockout of the autism gene CHD8 and characterization of its transcriptional networks in cerebral organoids derived from iPS cells. Molecular Autism. 2017;**8**:11